Gluten-Free One-Mix Baking

The Easy Way to Bake Without
Gluten, Dairy, or Soy

Diane M. Kuehn, PhD

Nutrition analysis by
Joan Nicholson, MA, CAS, RD, CDN, FAND, CHES

Copyright © 2020, 2018, 2014. Diane M. Kuehn. All rights reserved.

No portion of this work, in part or in the whole, may be copied, duplicated, broadcast, transmitted, or otherwise distributed without the written permission of the author.

ISBN-13: 978-1735527505

**Recipe testing by
The Brick House Cafe, Cicero, NY**

**Photographs by
Diane Kuehn and Sean Kuehn**

Deposited in the Library of Congress

Second Edition

Printed in the United States of America

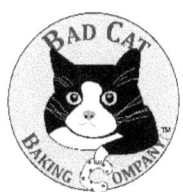

Bad Cat Baking Company LLC
Central Square, NY
badcatbakingcompany.com

Diane M. Kuehn *Gluten-Free One-Mix Baking*

Copyright © 2020, 2019, 2014, Diane M. Kuehn. All rights reserved.

No portion of this work, in part or in the whole, may be copied, duplicated, broadcast, transmitted, or otherwise distributed without the written permission of the author.

ISBN-13: 978-1-7337705

Recipe testing by
Mary Robyn Mackowiak, Glenmont, NY

Design work by
Michael Campisi and Sarah M. Jones

bat-Cat Baking Company, LLC
Capitol Region, NY
batcatbookprojects@gmail.com

Dedication

To Mark and Sean, the two best (and most honest) taste-testers! This book would not have been possible without your love and support.

Acknowledgements

Have you heard the expression "it takes a village to raise a child"? I've found that it takes a village to write a cookbook as well. Many thanks to the following in my village: Mark and Sean for sharing the gluten-free journey with me; my mom (a.k.a. Admiral Gluten) and dad for their encouragement; my mother-in-Law, Anne, for her editing skills and non-stop support; Laura, Joseph, Pam, both Bobs, Cole, Riley, Sara, and Emily for their support and willingness to eat my early gluten-free attempts; my friends, the Gordon, Kubis, Lowry, Martel, McLaughlin, Pennock, and Weber families for adapting so many meals for me; my dietary compadres, Brenda Wiseth and Diane Kiernan, for their willingness to listen and for making me realize that I am not alone when it comes to food sensitivities; Heather Engelman for her sensitivity to those with dietary concerns and for always providing a GF option at college events; Jane Nicholson for her non-stop enthusiasm for life and for connecting me with her mother, Joan; the Fabbioli family for letting me include Basil's wonderful family recipe for biscotti; the scouts and leaders of Boy Scout Troop 709 for providing honest feedback on my recipes and their efforts to keep gluten away from me on camp-outs (not a small feat); and Dr. Kaushal Nanavati and nutritionist Christine Carlson for teaching me so much about my own health and wellness.

This book would have not been possible without the knowledge and insight of the following people: Dr. Linda Lemay for her medical insight concerning this book and kindness throughout my healing process; Ginny Gordon for her friendship, non-stop encouragement, and willingness to test the recipes in her cafe (her suggestion about using vodka in the pie dough recipe is amazing); and Dr. Karen Magri and Terry Kirwan for their legal advice. I also extend thanks to my original publisher, Art Bell of Lexingford Publishing LLC (the first publisher of this book), who had faith in this project throughout. Finally, to Registered Dietitian, Joan Nicholson, thank you for your insight, knowledge, and support throughout the writing process -- this book would not have been possible without you!

Important Disclaimer

The contents of this cookbook are for informational purposes only and do not provide any medical advice. The contents of this book are not intended as a substitute for professional medical counsel, diagnosis, or treatment. Always seek the advice of your physician or other qualified health professional with any questions you have regarding a medical condition before making any major changes to your diet and before using any of the recipes or information in this book. Never disregard professional medical advice or delay in seeking it because of information you have read in this book. It is solely the reader's decision to use any of the recipes, information, or suggestions contained in this book. The author, consulting Registered Dietitian, and publisher are not responsible for any outcomes, results, or other consequences of the reader's use of the contents of this book. The author, consulting Registered Dietitian, and publisher do not recommend or endorse any specific medical tests, physicians, health care professionals, or products mentioned in this book. Always make sure that all the ingredients you use for these recipes are free of gluten, dairy, and soy, as well as any other items to which you are allergic or intolerant. It is important to note that some of the recipes in this book, although made with nutritious flours, can be high in calories, sugar, and saturated fat. Before making any recipe, consult with a professional healthcare professional to determine if these ingredients are suited to your health concerns and those of your family. The recipes in this book cannot be used for commercial purposes, without the expressed permission of the author.

About the Nutrition Analysis Used for this Book

The nutrition analysis information listed at the end of each recipe was estimated by Joan Nicholson, a Registered Dietician and Professor at the State University of New York at Morrisville, using The Food Processor® software version 10.12 by ESHA Research, Inc. (2013). This software bases its nutritional estimates on the USDA food composition tables.[1] Each recipe was analyzed for estimated caloric, carbohydrate, dietary fiber, sugar, protein, fat, dietary fiber, potassium, and sodium content. The nutrition analyses for recipes also include the percentages of other nutrients and minerals, such as iron and calcium, having percent daily values of 1% or more (based on a 2,000 calorie per day diet). Estimates are rounded to the nearest whole number.

Some other points are important to note concerning the nutrition data included in this cookbook. First, this nutrient content information should be used as a general guide only in consultation with your health professional, since results can vary from the estimates provided depending on the brands of ingredients used and accuracy of ingredient measurements. Second, if a choice of ingredients is given in a recipe (e.g., "shortening or lard"), the first ingredient listed is the one included in the nutrition analysis. Third, the estimates are based on the use of almond milk as the dairy-free "milk of choice," palm oil shortening as the shortening, and olive oil as the oil; using a different type of milk of choice, shortening, or oil will change the nutrient content. Fourth, the word "sugars" denotes all sugars (e.g., fructose, glucose, sucrose, and maltose) and includes the natural sugars found in fresh and dried fruit, as well as those in sweeteners such as honey, maple syrup, and cane sugar. Finally, any changes made to these recipes (including following any of the "Allergy/Intolerance Substitutions" or "Reduced Sugar" suggestions) will change the nutritional content of the baked goods from what is listed.

Table of Contents

Dedication	5
Acknowledgements	6
Important Disclaimer	8
Nutrition Analysis	9
Abbreviations and Conversions	14
Foreword	15
INTRODUCTION	17
Gluten-free Flour Mix Recipe	19
Ingredients in the Gluten-free Flour Mix	23
Baking without Gluten, Dairy, or Soy	42
Adapting the Recipes for Other Dietary Needs	52
Flour Substitutions	66
Do-it-yourself Ingredient Recipes	70
EASY BREAKFAST RECIPES	77
Granola	79
Pancakes	83
Waffles	87
Breakfast Cookies	91
Apple Oat Muffins	95
Lemon Almond Muffins	99
FRUIT AND VEGETABLE BREADS	103
Banana Chip Bread	105
Pumpkin Bread	109
Zucchini Bread	113
Carrot Spice Bread	117
Corn Bread with a Kick	121
Applesauce Oat Sandwich Bread	125
Home-style Poultry Stuffing	129

CAKES AND OTHER DESSERTS 133
Simple Yellow Cake 135
Rich Chocolate Cake 139
Moist Almond Crumb Cake 143
Blueberry Crumb Cake 147
Peach Upside-down Cake 151
Chocolate Chip Cake 155
Fresh Strawberry Cake 159
Maple Berry Crunch 163

BISCUIT, PIZZA, AND PIE DOUGHS 167
Basic Dinner Biscuits 169
Rosemary-Garlic Biscuits 173
Cranberry Orange Scones 177
Blueberry Scones 181
Pizza Dough 185
Single-crust Pie Dough 189
Double-crust Pie Dough 195

COOKIES AND TREATS 201
Chocolate Chip Cookies 203
Not-so-plain Sugar Cookies 207
Honey & Spice Cookies 211
Gingerbread Cookies 215
All-but-the-kitchen-sink Bars 219
Old-fashioned Oatmeal Cookies 223
Super Rich Brownies 227
Basil's Chocolate Biscotti 231
"Butter" Cookies 235
Fried Dough 239

TOPPINGS, SIDES, AND FROSTINGS	243
Cashew-Coconut Cream Topping	245
Chocolate Coconut Ganache or Frosting	249
Vanilla Frosting	253
Lemon-, Orange-, or Vanilla-flavored Icing	255
Frozen Coconut Vanilla Custard	257
Coconut Yogurt	261
REFERENCES	267
INDEX	275

Abbreviations and Conversions

Common Abbreviations:

GF	Gluten-free
DF	Dairy-free
SF	Soy-free
c.	Cup
T.	Tablespoon
t.	Teaspoon
oz.	Ounce
g	Gram
ml	Milliliter
l	Liter
F	Fahrenheit
C	Celsius

Some useful conversions:

1 Tablespoon = 3 teaspoons
¼ cup = 4 Tablespoons
1 quart = 0.95 liters
1 ounce = 28.3 grams
Oven temperatures: 375° F = 191° C; 350° F = 177° C; 325° F = 163° C

Foreword

Food sensitivities and allergies are never easy to deal with, especially in a society that loves fast food and pre-packaged treats. For those of us who deal with dietary challenges every day, making nutritious and delicious goodies at home—foods that make both our bodies and taste buds happy—is essential.

The delicious recipes that I share here with you were created after I was diagnosed with gluten sensitivity in 2008. In later years, as my auto-immune problems triggered intolerances to dairy, soy, eggs, canola oil, and histamine-rich foods, I began adapting the recipes for my new sensitivities. The final touch to this book came thanks to Registered Dietitian Joan Nicholson. Through Joan's extensive knowledge and support, the nutrition analyses for the recipes were added. With Joan, I began to rethink portion size and ingredients, and realized that every bite of food—especially for those with food intolerances—needs to be packed full of nutrition and taste.

Writing this book has given me the chance to explore the incredible diversity of vitamin-rich ingredients available to those of us who wish to make healthful food choices. These recipes combine nutrition, taste, and quick preparation. By using a single gluten-free flour mix, prep time for most of the recipes in this book is about fifteen minutes (not including baking time). Because the flour mix includes a variety of flours and starches, those that are not compatible with specific health concerns can be easily switched out with little to no change in the final product

(I've included suggestions throughout this book to make these substitutions easy).

I hope you enjoy these recipes as much as I've enjoyed creating them. I wish you healthy—and delicious—eating!

Introduction

About the Gluten-free Flour Mix...

This flour mix is the result of four years of experimentation, many failed baking attempts, and much patience on the part of my family. The result is a gluten-, dairy-, and soy-free flour mixture that makes great-tasting baked goods rich in flavor and nutrition. The recipes in this book are not designed to be gourmet recipes; rather, they are easy, tasty recipes suitable for family meals and desserts. Do not expect these recipes to taste like those made from bleached wheat flour; the baked goods made with this book are much richer in flavor due to the nutrients in the whole grain flours used. It is important to note that the recipes provided here may not be suitable for everyone. Those with special dietary needs should consult their doctor or nutritionist before using these recipes or adapting them to their diets.

The flour mix used in this book is different from store-bought gluten-free flour mixes in several ways:

1. Nutrition. This flour mix is more nutritious than most store-bought gluten-free mixes which often contain a high percentage of white rice flour and some type of starch. Although starch is necessary in gluten-free flour mixes, it is relatively easy to replace the white rice flour with more nutritious flours such as brown rice, millet, and sorghum. These whole grain flours boost the nutritional value of the mix, an important consideration for those with food allergies and intolerances.

2. One mix. Using only one flour mix means that you can make many baked goods (including pancakes and biscuits) easily. Using multiple flour mixes clogs up pantry space and can be time consuming to make. Using one gluten-free flour mix eliminates these problems. While most of the recipes in this book are based on this one flour mix, several recipes require the addition of extra flours or starches to achieve the best results.

3. Less time. The flour mix takes about five minutes to prepare. The only time-consuming part of making the mix may be purchasing the different flours that go into it. All of the flours are readily available in the gluten-free section of large grocery stores, natural food stores, online, or in Asian grocery stores (a source for sweet rice flour and some starches). No matter their source, be sure that all of the flours you use are free of gluten and any other allergens of concern. Once the mix is made, most of the recipes in this book take about 15 minutes to prepare (not including baking time).

4. Easy to adapt to dietary needs. The diversity of flours and starches used in the gluten-free flour mix makes it easy to adapt to your specific dietary needs. If you cannot tolerate a specific type of flour, simply switch it for a flour that you can tolerate. Buckwheat and amaranth flours are good alternatives that make only a slight difference in the taste and texture of the recipes. Teff flour is also a good substitute, but can make baked goods slightly denser in consistency. Avoid using nut or seed meals (e.g., almond meal, flax meal), corn meal or flour, or additional rice flour as substitutes since your baked goods may become gritty in texture. Using fava or garbanzo bean flour is also not recommended as a substitute since it can make your baked goods dense in texture. Suitable substitutions are discussed in the "Flour Substitutions" section of this book.

5. Less expensive. Making the gluten-free flour mix yourself costs about half the price of buying a pre-made gluten-free mix of equal quality and nutritional content. If you do decide to use a store-bought brand for these recipes, make sure to find a nutritious one that includes diverse flours other than just white rice flour and a starch.

Gluten-Free Flour Mix Recipe

Most gluten-free flour mixes use a flour-to-starch ratio that is roughly 1:1. The ratio of the mix below favors the flours slightly, boosting the nutritional value and dietary fiber content of the mix. All of the flours and starches needed for this mix are easily found in large supermarkets or natural foods stores. The sweet rice flour (also called mochiko or "glutinous" rice flour, though it does not naturally contain gluten) can also be found in Asian supermarkets. If you live far from a large supermarket, online sources will ship the flours and starches right to your door.

Always check all your flours and starches (as well as other recipe ingredients) to make sure they are free of gluten and any other allergens of concern. Depending on your level of sensitivity, you may also need to make sure that your ingredients do not contain trace amounts of allergens (e.g., some brands of GF flours and starches contain traces of soy and/or tree nuts due to their production on shared equipment). If you are intolerant of any of the flours or starches in the mix, simply switch them out for flours or starches that you do tolerate (see Table 1 for flour and starch substitution suggestions). Some flours not to use as replacements in this flour mix are corn flour or meal, nut or seed meals, bean flour, or coconut flour. Note that this flour mix does not include baking powder because of its short shelf-life. This recipe makes nearly 7 cups.

☑ Allergy/Intolerance Substitutions:

All: Xanthan gum is produced from sugars derived from wheat, dairy, soy, or corn. Check with the manufacturer to determine if the brand you choose is free of your allergens of concern. Use guar gum as a substitute if needed, or leave out completely if you cannot find a safe brand.

Rice: Replace the brown rice flour with an equal measure of amaranth flour, and replace the sweet rice flour (which is more similar to a starch than a flour) with an equal measure of arrowroot starch or tapioca starch.

Nightshade family: Use either arrowroot starch or tapioca starch in place of potato starch.

Histamine: Do not use buckwheat flour as a substitute for other flours. If potato starch is not tolerated, replace it with either arrowroot starch or tapioca starch (if tolerated). Leave out the xanthan and guar gums if not tolerated (no replacement; your final baked goods may be slightly crumbly). Be sure to check with your medical practitioner concerning the use of all ingredients in this flour mix.

Salicylates: Do not use corn flour, corn starch, corn meal, almond meal, or other nut meals as a substitute for other flours. If potato starch is not tolerated, replace it with either arrowroot starch or tapioca starch (if tolerated). If sorghum flour is not tolerated, replace it with either amaranth or quinoa flour as tolerated. Leave out the xanthan and guar gums if not tolerated (no replacement; your final baked goods may be slightly crumbly). Be sure to check with your medical practitioner concerning the use of all ingredients in this flour mix.

Ingredients:
1 c. sorghum flour (120 g)
1 c. brown or white rice flour (120 g)
1 c. sweet (glutinous) rice flour or other finely-ground rice flour (should be the texture of corn starch; 120 g)
1 c. millet flour (136 g)
2⅔ c. starch (arrowroot, potato, or tapioca starch; 328 g)
4 t. baking soda (20 g)
2 T. xanthan gum or guar gum (20 g)

Directions:
Step 1. Measure the ingredients by scooping with the appropriate measuring cup or spoon, and leveling off with the flat edge of a knife, or by weighing. Place the ingredients in a gallon-sized zipper bag. Seal the bag tightly and shake till the ingredients are well combined.

Step 2. Make sure to shake the bag to re-combine the ingredients before each use. Because of the heaviness of gluten-free flours, sifting the flour mix prior to use generally does not make a noticeable difference in the finished product.

Nutritional content: Makes 7 servings (1 cup (148 g) per serving). Each serving contains: Calories (500); Total Fat (1.5 g); Saturated Fat (0 g); Cholesterol (0 mg); Sodium (720 mg.); Potassium (105 mg); Total Carbohydrate (118 g); Dietary Fiber (5 g); Sugars (1 g); Protein (6 g). Nutrient(s) of note (percent of Daily Value): Iron 15% DV

Ingredients in the Gluten-free Flour Mix

The ingredients used in this flour mix provide many of the vitamins and minerals needed on a daily basis. Most of the flours (in comparison to the starches) are high in protein and dietary fiber. Make sure that all of the ingredients you use are free of any allergens to which you may be sensitive. If you are unsure if a brand of flour or starch is free of gluten, dairy, and soy or other allergens, check directly with the manufacturer before use.

Arrowroot Starch

Vitamins and minerals: Moderate source of calcium, iron, folate, and manganese.[2]

Other facts: Arrowroot starch (also called arrowroot flour) is a fine powder made from the thick tubers (roots) of the arrowroot plant (*Maranta arundinacea*). A native of South America, arrowroot is cultivated today in South America, the Caribbean, and the Philippines. This starch is known for its ability to be digested easily.[3]

Why it's needed in the gluten-free flour mix: All gluten-free flour mixes are roughly half starch and half flour. While the flour half contributes to the nutritional value of the mix, the starch contributes to the light texture of baked goods and, in some cases, crispness. Starch also mellows the flavor of the gluten-free flours, some of which can be strong tasting. Potato starch or tapioca starch can be used in place of arrowroot starch for recipes.

Baking Soda

<u>Vitamins and minerals:</u> Negligible amounts.

<u>Other facts:</u> Baking soda is sodium bicarbonate that is created by combining carbonic acid with sodium hydroxide.[4] Baking soda is the source of the sodium listed in the nutritional content of the gluten-free flour mix recipe.

<u>Why it's needed in the gluten-free flour mix:</u> Baking soda makes baked goods rise. You'll notice that it is included in the gluten-free flour mix instead of baking powder (although baking powder is included in many of the recipes in this book). Baking soda does not deteriorate as quickly as baking powder, and so is a more stable leavening (rising) agent to have in the gluten-free flour mix (especially if you store the mix longer than a few weeks). It also releases carbon dioxide bubbles into your batter, making baked goods light and airy.

Brown Rice Flour

<u>Vitamins and minerals:</u> High in niacin, thiamin, B6, and pantothenic acid. Good source of iron, phosphorus, magnesium, manganese, selenium, and zinc.[5]

<u>Other facts:</u> Brown rice flour was first cultivated in China an estimated 6,000 to 9,000 years ago. Due to trade routes through the Middle East and Europe, rice eventually made its way west. Brown rice flour, which contains the nutritious outer hull of the rice grain, is much higher in vitamins and minerals than white rice flour which has had the outer hull removed.[6] Recent studies, however, have

found that trace amounts of naturally-occurring inorganic arsenic (i.e., arsenic found in the soil) are found in rice. Brown rice in particular often contains more arsenic than white rice since arsenic tends to accumulate in the outer hull of the rice grain. Inorganic arsenic is a concern because it is a carcinogen.[7] Eating large quantities of rice could in particular be a concern for infants because of their small body weight. In 2016, the U.S. Food and Drug Administration proposed a limit on the amount of inorganic arsenic allowed in infant rice cereal (100 parts per billion).[8] Monitor how much rice you use each week. If you eat rice frequently, you may wish to switch the brown rice flour used in the flour mix recipe for a different type of flour such as amaranth or buckwheat, or use white rice flour instead which is usually lower in inorganic arsenic.

Why it's needed in the gluten-free flour mix: Brown rice flour gives your baked goods structure, allowing cakes and breads to rise without falling upon cooling. Don't use more than the amount shown in the gluten-free flour mix recipe, though — too much will make your baked goods gritty in texture.

Guar Gum

Vitamins and minerals: Negligible amounts.

Other facts: Guar gum is a powder made from the dried seeds of the guar plant (*Cyamopsis tetragonoloba*), a native of the Middle East.[9]

Why it's needed in the gluten-free flour mix: Guar gum serves the same purpose as xanthan gum — to bind together ingredients and keep gluten-free baked goods from crumbling. Guar gum is not made using corn (like some brands of xanthan gum) and so is often used by those with corn allergies.

Millet Flour

<u>Vitamins and minerals:</u> High in niacin, thiamin, riboflavin, B6, and folate. Good source of iron, phosphorous, magnesium, zinc, copper, and manganese.[10]

<u>Other facts:</u> Another of the ancient grains, millet originated in Northern Africa. Evidence suggests that it was used during prehistoric times as a food source. Although it's a common ingredient in bird seed, its use as a food source for humans is increasing in the United States.[11]

<u>Why it's needed in the gluten-free flour mix:</u> Millet, like sorghum, gives baked goods a springy texture and helps retain moisture in the final product.

Potato Starch

<u>Vitamins and minerals:</u> Good source of resistant starch ("resists" digestion in the intestine, supporting the growth of healthy bacteria in the colon).[12]

<u>Other facts:</u> Potatoes are members of the Solanaceae or nightshade family, a group of plants that includes tomatoes and eggplants. Potato starch is not the same as potato flour, which is made from whole dried potatoes that are ground; the starch is instead extracted from crushed potatoes through a washing process, and then dried.

Why it's needed in the gluten-free flour mix: As with other starches, potato starch works to lighten the taste and texture of gluten-free baked goods. Replacing the potato starch with arrowroot starch or tapioca starch works well in these recipes.

Sweet Rice Flour (White or Brown)

Vitamins and minerals: Moderate amounts of niacin and thiamin. Good source of manganese and selenium.[13]

Other facts: Also called sticky rice, mochiko, or glutinous rice (though it does not contain gluten), this type of rice has been cultivated in Asia specifically for its sticky texture.

Why it's needed in the gluten-free flour mix: Sweet rice flour (a very finely ground rice flour) is essential to this flour mix -- do not replace it with regular brown or white rice flour. Unlike regular rice flour (which can make baked goods gritty), sweet rice flour gives baked goods a light and smooth texture. Although *white* sweet rice flour gives a smoother consistency to baked goods than does *brown* sweet rice flour, brown sweet rice flour may contain higher levels of nutrients (and possibly inorganic arsenic as well) since it includes the hull of the rice grain. White sweet rice flour is available from certain manufacturers in the United States (e.g., Bob's Red Mill®, Koda Farms®) or Asian food stores (I often use a glutinous rice flour from Thailand -- a country where little wheat is grown). Always check the source of the sweet rice flour you choose to make sure it is free of any allergens of concern.

Sorghum Flour

<u>Vitamins and minerals:</u> High in niacin, thiamin, and riboflavin. Good source of iron, phosphorus and potassium.[14]

<u>Other facts:</u> Sorghum originated in northern Africa, and was domesticated for human consumption in either northern Africa or India. Thought to have been brought to the United States by enslaved Africans, sorghum is the fifth largest cereal crop in the world today.[15]

<u>Why it's needed in the gluten-free flour mix:</u> Sorghum gives a slightly nutty flavor to the flour mix that is not overpowering. It also gives your baked goods a springy texture.

Tapioca Starch

<u>Vitamins and minerals:</u> Contains a small amount of iron.[16]

<u>Other facts</u>: Tapioca starch is a fine white powder made from the roots of the Cassava plant (*Manihot esculenta*), a native of South America. Tapioca is now cultivated worldwide.[17]

<u>Why it's needed in the gluten-free flour mix:</u> As with other starches, tapioca starch works to lighten the taste and texture of gluten-free baked goods. With its slightly sweet flavor, tapioca starch works well in dessert recipes. Potato starch or arrowroot starch can be used in place of tapioca starch for these recipes.

Xanthan Gum

Vitamins and minerals: Negligible amounts.

Other facts: Xanthan gum is a powder produced by the *Xanthomonas campestris* bacteria as it digests *sugars* derived from corn, wheat, soy, or milk.[18] Because wheat protein (i.e., gluten) is not normally used to make xanthan gum, certain brands of xanthan gum made from wheat sugars are certified as gluten-free according to the U.S. Food and Drug Administration's guidelines for gluten content. Milk sugar (lactose) is also often used to make xanthan gum. Check with the manufacturer of the brand you choose to make sure it is free of your allergens of concern. Those with extreme sensitivities to wheat, soy, milk, or corn may wish to avoid using xanthan gum. If the manufacturer cannot guarantee that it is safe for your allergies, leave it out completely or use guar gum instead.

Why it's needed in the gluten-free flour mix: Xanthan gum binds together the ingredients in gluten-free baked goods. Without this additive, baked goods may be slightly crumbly.

Other Common Ingredients Used in this Cookbook

For all ingredients listed in this cookbook, check with the manufacturers to make sure they are certified as free of gluten, dairy, and soy, as well as any other allergens of concern.

Almonds and Almond Meal

<u>Vitamins and minerals:</u> High in protein, fiber, and healthy fats, almonds also contain calcium, magnesium, copper, potassium, and vitamin E.[19]

<u>Other facts:</u> Thought to come from China and Central Asia, almond trees were brought west to Southern Europe on the Silk Road during the Middle Ages. In the 1700s, they were brought to California from Spain by the Franciscans.[20] Today, almonds are an important crop in California. When purchasing almonds and almond meal, make sure to purchase a brand that is gluten-free (this applies to all types of nuts in general); many manufacturers inadvertently add trace amounts of gluten to their nuts during processing.

<u>Why it's needed in recipes:</u> Almond meal gives recipes a sweet taste, and also keeps baked goods moist. If you have a tree nut allergy, almonds, almond extract, almond milk, and almond meal should not be used in recipes; substitutions for almond-based ingredients are given throughout this book. Almond milk is one option for the "milk of choice" included in some of the recipes, and is used to calculate the nutrition content estimates contained in this book. Use a different type of non-dairy

milk if you are concerned about the fat that almond milk contains or if you are sensitive to tree nuts.

Baking Powder

<u>Vitamins and minerals:</u> Negligible amounts.

<u>Other facts:</u> Baking powder is often a mixture of sodium bicarbonate, sodium aluminum sulfate, monocalcium phosphate, and some type of starch (usually either corn or potato starch). Double-acting baking powder is recommended for these recipes since it will give your batter some rise immediately (as the dough is being mixed), and then again during the baking process.

<u>Why it's needed in recipes:</u> Baking powder makes it possible for gluten-free cakes and muffins to rise. If you notice that your baked goods are not rising adequately, the problem may be that an old can of baking powder is being used. After a can has been opened, baking powder rapidly deteriorates. Replace a can of baking powder after it has been open for more than two months. Individuals sensitive to corn or potatoes should choose a brand that does not contain these starches.

Chia Seeds

<u>Vitamins and minerals:</u> High in fiber and protein, chia seeds are a good source of calcium, manganese, phosphorous, and omega-3 and omega-6 fatty acids.[21]

<u>Other facts:</u> The tiny, black chia seed comes from the *Salvia hispanica* plant, a member of the mint family. Grown in Central and South America, chia seeds are

thought to have been used historically by the ancient Aztecs and Mayans.[22]

Why it's needed in recipes: Though mild in flavor, chia seeds add a wonderful texture and crunch to baked goods. Because they form a thick gel when placed in a liquid, chia seeds work well as an egg substitute and as a thickener for soups and jams.

Coconut Milk

Vitamins and minerals: Rich in medium-chain fatty acids, protein, magnesium, manganese, iron, phosphorous, zinc, and folate, and cholesterol free.[23]

Other facts: Coconut is the fruit of the coconut palm, a native of the South Pacific islands and Polynesia.[24] When a coconut is split open, coconut meat and coconut water are found inside. Pulverizing the coconut meat makes coconut butter (also called creamed coconut or cream of coconut) and releases coconut oil. Coconut milk is a creamy liquid made by mixing together water and the flesh of the coconut. Coconut cream is the thick, creamy layer that forms when coconut milk is refrigerated overnight.[25] Coconut flour is coconut meat that has been dried and ground into a fine powder. Coconut contains lauric acid, a medium-chain fatty acid (the source of the saturated fat in coconut) thought to increase HDL ("good") cholesterol and help with digestion.[26] However, the high saturated fat content of coconut may not be suitable for everyone; consult with a licensed medical practitioner before adding coconut to your diet.

Why it's needed in recipes: Coconut cream and coconut milk are often used as replacements for dairy. They provide a richness to recipes that is hard to beat (even by dairy). If you use *canned* whole-fat coconut milk as the "milk of choice" in a recipe, recombine the coconut cream with the coconut water prior to use by gently warming it, and then add water to thin it to the consistency of whole-fat cow's milk (a ratio of 1 cup canned coconut milk to 1 cup water works well). Canned "lite" coconut milk and homemade coconut milk (see the "Do-it-yourself Ingredient Recipes" section of this book) do not need to be thinned prior to use in these recipes. For the frosting and ganache recipes in this book, full-fat coconut milk in a BPA-free can or Tetra Pak® is recommended; the thicker consistency of the cream in the store-bought coconut milk will give you better results than using "lite" or homemade coconut milk.

Eggs

Vitamins and minerals: High in protein, cholesterol, omega-3 fatty acids (depending on the diet of the chickens), omega-6 fatty acids, and many vitamins and nutrients (vitamins A, D, and E, B-vitamins, folate, pantothenic acid, selenium, phosphorous, iron, zinc, calcium, lutein, and choline are some).[27]

Other facts: Cutting eggs from the diet has long been viewed as a way to reduce LDL ("bad") cholesterol levels and improve heart health. However, except for those with certain health conditions like diabetes, eggs used in moderation may have a minimal impact on blood cholesterol levels.[28] In addition, the high degree of nutrients in eggs may be beneficial for some individuals. It is important to discuss the benefits and potential health risks of eating eggs with your medical practitioner. If you do decide to bake with eggs, look for eggs from pasture-raised chickens fed an organic diet.

Why it's needed in recipes: Eggs work as an important binder, keeping cakes from crumbling, pie dough flakey, and crumb toppings crisp. Eggs also help with the lightness of baked goods. Egg replacers can be used in most of the recipes for those who are vegan, have egg allergies or intolerances, or with cholesterol or other health concerns (see the egg replacer recipes in the "Do-it-yourself Ingredient Recipes" section on page 73). The recipes in this book have been created using large eggs; you may get inconsistent results if you use eggs that are jumbo, extra-large, medium, or small.

Flax Meal

Vitamins and minerals: High in omega-3 and omega-6 fatty acids, as well as protein and fiber. Excellent source of manganese, magnesium, phosphorous, copper, thiamin, calcium, iron, and zinc.[29]

Other facts: Flax (*Linum usitatissimum*) is one of the most versatile plants. With human use dating back to the Ancient Egyptians (when it was used to create linen), different varieties of flax are still used today for fiber to make linens, seeds for human and animal consumption (it is an important food source for livestock and pets), and to make linseed oil. Omega-3 eggs are produced by feeding flax seed to chickens.[30]

Why it's needed in recipes: Flax meal helps boost the nutrients and protein in many different types of baked goods. It stabilizes breads and muffins, and provides a hearty texture. It is an excellent egg substitute when mixed with water, but may not be suitable for those with a histamine or salicylate intolerance, or other digestive system problems.

Honey

Vitamins and minerals: Rich in vitamin B6, niacin, riboflavin, calcium, iron, manganese, copper, magnesium, potassium, and zinc. [31]

Other facts: Honey was used as the primary sweetener in Europe before granulated sugar made from sugar cane was brought to Europe via trade routes from the east. Far more nutritious than granulated cane sugar, honey contains both fructose ("fruit sugar") and glucose[32]— monosaccharide sugars that may be easier for sensitive digestive systems to break down. Honey should not be given to children younger than one year of age since it may contain the spores of bacteria that can cause rare but fatal reactions in infants.

Why it's needed in recipes: Honey gives a sweetness to baked goods. For most of the recipes in this book, the cane sugar can be replaced with an equivalent amount of honey. When using honey in place of sugar, however, you may notice that your baked goods will not rise quite as well; the increase in nutritional value makes up for this slight difference in rise. Do not replace the sugar in crumb toppings, frostings, or icings with honey.

Lard

<u>Vitamins and minerals:</u> Negligible.

<u>Other facts:</u> When pork fat is melted down (i.e., rendered), filtered, and clarified, "processed" lard is produced. "Leaf lard" (made from the fat surrounding the kidneys and loin of the pig) is considered the highest quality type of lard, but, depending on where you live, may not be readily available.[33] If you decide to cook with lard, choose an organic, un-hydrogenated brand that has been minimally processed and is preservative free. Some manufacturers hydrogenate lard during the processing which makes it stable at room temperature, but adds trans fats; some brands contain preservatives as well. Though unprocessed lard contains less saturated fat than butter[34], it may not be a viable option for those with certain health conditions, and is not suitable for vegans or vegetarians.

<u>Why it's needed in recipes:</u> Lard keeps baked goods moist, but also contributes to a light texture. For pies, lard creates a flaky crust.

Milk of Choice

<u>Vitamins and minerals:</u> Varies by type of milk chosen.

<u>Other facts:</u> Different types of dairy-free milk are readily available in most grocery stores today, and can be used interchangeably in these recipes. Types of milks to consider are almond, hemp, rice, hazelnut, and coconut. It is important to read the labels on non-dairy milk products because many contain preservatives and thickeners that may not be suitable for some individuals (e.g., those with a

histamine intolerance may be intolerant of carrageenan, a thickener sometimes used in non-dairy milk products).

Why it's needed in recipes: Nut, seed, and rice milks add a creaminess to recipes, and also help your baked goods rise. Recipes for making your own nut or rice milks are found in the "Do-it-yourself Ingredient Recipes" section (page 70). It is important to realize that you may get different results for your baked goods based on the water content of the milk you use; choose a non-dairy milk that is the consistency of whole-fat cow's milk for best results. Cow's milk can be used as the "milk of choice" in the recipes in this book for those who are not dairy intolerant.

Oats (Certified Gluten-Free Only)

Vitamins and minerals: High in protein and fiber, oats also contain folate, magnesium, potassium, and phosphorous.[35]

Other facts: It is not known where the cultivation of oats as a crop originated, but oats have been used for food as far back as 2000 BC in Egypt. Today, oats are mainly grown in Europe and North America.[36] Due to the shared milling process of oats, barley, and wheat in the United States, most brands of oats contain gluten. Purchase and use only "certified" gluten-free rolled oats for the recipes in this cookbook; do not use quick cooking oats. Some brands of certified gluten-free oats are produced in facilities that also process other allergens such as soy and tree nuts; check with the manufacturer to make sure the brand of oats you choose is suited to your health concerns. Also, make sure the oats you buy have not been repackaged; some bulk food stores will repackage certified gluten-free oats, inadvertently adding gluten to a product that was originally gluten-free. Finally, if you do not tolerate oats, skip the recipes in this book that contain oats or follow the substitution suggestions in the recipe.

<u>Why it's needed in recipes:</u> Gluten-free rolled oats give recipes a nutty, hearty texture that works well in granola, crumb toppings, and some cookies. Oat flour helps to stabilize the texture of sandwich bread. You can easily make your own oat flour by pulsing certified gluten-free rolled oats in a food processor till a flour forms.

Pure Olive Oil (NOT Extra Virgin)

<u>Vitamins and minerals:</u> Good source of vitamins E and K, and omega-3 and omega-6 fatty acids.[37]

<u>Other facts:</u> For most people, olive oil is one of the healthiest oils you can use in baked goods and for cooking in general. While extra virgin olive oil gives salads a wonderful flavor and is great for sautéing, its strong olive flavor can overpower your baked goods and its low smoke point can cause deep-fried foods to burn. Look for a "pure" olive oil that is *not* extra virgin (i.e., not from the first press) to prevent these problems.

<u>Why it's needed in recipes:</u> Olive oil helps retain moisture in baked goods, and also prevents them from sticking to the pan. The olive oil used in the recipes in this book can be replaced with another neutral-flavored oil (but not butter, lard, or shortening) if needed. Those with a salicylate intolerance should not use olive oil.

Quinoa Flour

Vitamins and minerals: High in protein, 20 amino acids, fiber, and many nutrients including manganese, magnesium, phosphorous, folate, copper, iron, and thiamine.[38]

Other facts: Quinoa flour is made by grinding the tiny seeds of the *Chenopodium quinoa* plant. The use of quinoa for human consumption dates back to about 5,000 years ago in the Andes Mountains of South America, where it was considered a sacred crop by the Incas.[39] Today, quinoa is considered one of the healthiest "grain-like" ingredients available due to its complete protein profile and diverse nutrients.[40]

Why it's needed in recipes: Quinoa is an excellent flour to use when you want to increase the protein content of a recipe. Too much of this nutritious flour, however, can make baked goods taste slightly bitter.

Shortening

Vitamins and minerals: Negligible for most brands.

Other facts: Vegetarians and vegans will want to use shortening instead of lard in the recipes in this book. Make sure to always check the ingredients in shortenings — only a few brands are gluten, dairy, and soy free. In addition, some contain canola oil to which some people are sensitive. Use only a non-hydrogenated shortening (e.g., Spectrum®, a palm oil-based shortening). Hydrogenated shortenings (including some solid brands of margarine) have had the fatty acids in them chemically-altered to extend the shelf life of the product, increasing the amount of "trans fats" they contain. Trans fats have been shown to increase LDL ("bad") cholesterol levels, and have been linked to heart disease, stroke, and diabetes.[41] If you tolerate dairy, the shortening in the recipes can be replaced with butter.

Why it's needed in recipes: Shortening keeps baked goods moist, contributes to a crisp texture, and keeps baked goods from sticking to the pan.

Stevia

Vitamins and minerals: Negligible.

Other facts: Stevia is an extract made from the leaves of the *Stevia rebaudiana* plant. Though 30 times sweeter than sugar, stevia has a negligible effect on blood glucose levels.[42] Little is currently known about the potential side effects of stevia, so check with your medical practitioner to make sure stevia is safe for you before adding it to any recipe. If your medical practitioner approves replacing sugars with stevia, use a brand of clear, alcohol-free liquid stevia that does not contain additives other than water and glycerin (e.g., NuNaturals®). Many brands of powdered stevia contain fillers and additives that some individuals may not tolerate. Liquid stevia that is brown or green in color may have a bitter aftertaste, so use a clear liquid stevia. Though a small bottle of clear liquid stevia may be expensive, one bottle can last for up to six months, depending on how often it is used.

Why it's needed in recipes: Stevia is used as a sugar-free replacement for natural and processed sugars. Many of the recipes in this cookbook come out well when the sugars are replaced with clear, alcohol-free liquid stevia. The concentration of stevia often differs between brands; depending on your taste, you may need to add more or less stevia than is directed in each recipe. Getting the amount of stevia correct can be a challenge since relatively little is needed. A trick I use (particularly for batters containing raw egg) is to put together the batter, mix in the amount of liquid stevia recommended in the recipe, place a spoonful of the batter on a plate, and microwave it till cooked (usually about 30-40 seconds). Once cooled, you can safely taste the cooked batter to see if the level of stevia is adequate; add more stevia if needed.

Sugar (Refined Cane)

Vitamins and minerals: Negligible.

Other facts: Sugar has been produced from sugarcane for thousands of years. Originally from Polynesia, the use of cane sugar spread to Asia and the Middle East, and then eventually to Europe. The process of extracting cane juice from the sugar cane plant and then evaporating the juice to form granulated sugar was developed in India about 500 BC.[43] Unfortunately, any nutrients found in the sugar cane plant are removed during processing. Cane sugar is made of sucrose (a disaccharide comprised of fructose and glucose) which must be broken down in the digestive system in order to be absorbed.[44]

Why it's needed in recipes: Cane sugar adds sweetness to cakes and cookies, and supports the structure of baked goods (it prevents them from collapsing upon cooling). If you wish to use honey or clear liquid, alcohol-free stevia in place of cane sugar for the recipes in this book, you may notice a change in the outcome of the recipes (e.g., cakes might not rise or brown as well, and cookie dough may be a little harder to work with). "Reduced sugar" directions are given for many of the recipes in this book.

Baking without Gluten, Dairy, or Soy

Avoiding Allergens in Store-Bought Ingredients

The U.S. Food and Drug Administration (FDA) requires that any packaged foods regulated by the FDA for sale in the United States clearly list on their ingredients label if they contain any of the eight major food allergens: milk, soy, wheat, eggs, tree nuts, peanuts, shellfish, and fish. Because gluten, rye, and barley are not required to be specified, a product can be labeled as "wheat free" but still not be gluten-free.[45] Although the FDA does require manufacturers to identify if trace amounts of the eight major allergens above are present in their products, it is often difficult to know if trace amounts of other allergens such as rye, barley, or corn are present. In addition, incorrect product labeling for the eight major allergens can occur. Depending on your level of sensitivity, you may need to use products that are completely free of your allergens of concern and produced in a facility where these allergens are not used at all. Check product labels each time you purchase an item to make sure the manufacturer has not changed the ingredients used or the processing. If you are unsure about a product, call the manufacturer to make sure it does not contain the allergens of concern, that its ingredients are not derived from your allergens of concern, and that it is not made on equipment "shared" with allergen-containing products. More details about what to look for on product labels specifically for gluten, dairy, and soy are given below; information on other allergens (such as corn) is included in the "Adapting the recipes for other dietary needs" section on page 52.

Avoiding Gluten

According to the FDA, items can be labeled as "gluten-free" in the United States if they are below 20 ppm in gluten content[46]; however, it is still unclear if this standard is adequate for extremely sensitive individuals or those with Celiac's Disease. The best way to avoid gluten completely is by carefully reading and understanding the fine print on product labels. Some pointers to look for before purchasing products are:

- Check to see if wheat, rye, or barley, as well as ingredients derived from wheat, rye, or barley, are listed as ingredients. Some ingredients (e.g., maltodextrin, dextrin) can be derived from wheat as well as from gluten-free grains such as corn. Contact the manufacturer to find out more about the ingredients in a product before purchasing it.
- Avoid using flours, starches, and other ingredients (e.g., spices, flavored extracts, and non-dairy milk products) that are produced in a facility where gluten-containing products are made, unless you know for certain that the manufacturer tests the product for gluten and uses special precautions to separate the processing of gluten-containing and gluten-free products. Manufacturers will sometimes indicate if products are made on "shared" or "separate" equipment.

- Don't purchase a product just because it states "gluten-free" on the label. Always check the fine print to see if the item is completely without gluten, or if it contains trace amounts below 20 ppm. If you are unsure, call the manufacturer; most manufacturers in the U. S. today are able to provide this information for their customers. Many larger manufacturers also post their policy online with regard to the gluten labeling of their products.
- Know the names of the various types of wheat (e.g., kamut, durum, semolina, spelt, triticale, farro, emmer, einkorn, triticum, graham) as these are sometimes listed on ingredient labels.
- Look for other sources of gluten such as barley, rye, malt, and malt vinegar since items advertised as "wheat free" may not be "gluten-free" (i.e., they may contain barley or rye).
- When choosing alcoholic beverages, choose beers brewed only from gluten-free grains such as sorghum (beers that have been "filtered" to remove gluten may contain trace amounts of gluten). Avoid malted beverages as these are made from barley. "Flavored" liquors may also contain gluten.
- Finally, verify that ingredients such as extracts or "flavorings," food colors or dyes, preservatives, and other additives are gluten-free.

Avoiding Dairy

For a dairy allergy or sensitivity, it is important to know if you are sensitive to lactose, a sugar found in milk; allergic or sensitive to casein, a protein found in milk; and/or allergic or sensitive to whey, another protein found in milk. Individuals with a lactose intolerance alone may be able to enjoy "lactose free" products such as lactose free milk, while those with a casein or whey intolerance or allergy need to avoid dairy completely.[47] Avoid products containing ingredients such as milk, cream, yogurt, butter, ghee, cheese, lactose, casein or caseinate, curds, and whey, as well as products derived from these ingredients. Some additional tips for those with a dairy sensitivity are:

- Read the ingredient labels of products carefully. Be cautious of items that state they are "lactose free" or "dairy free" as these may contain casein; similarly, items that state they are "casein free" may contain lactose.
- Carefully read the ingredient list of products such as "dairy free" cheeses, mayonnaise, and tuna fish as they may contain casein.
- Know if the ingredients in a product are derived from dairy. For example, xanthan gum can be produced from lactose, as well as from sugars derived from wheat, corn, or soy.
- Check with the manufacturer of a product if you are unsure if the product contains dairy, or has been derived from dairy.

Avoiding Soy

Soy from soy beans, frequently referred to as soya outside of the United States, is used to make many products including soy oil, soy lecithin, soy protein, tofu, natto, tempeh, soy milk, miso, soy flour, soy sauce, and teriyaki sauce. Some tips for avoiding soy are:

- Know if you tolerate soy lecithin and soy oil before buying any product. Some (but not all) individuals with a soy intolerance tolerate soy lecithin and soy

oil because of the minimal amount of soy protein these products contain. However, the amount of protein in soy lecithin and soy oil can differ between brands so use caution if choosing any product containing these ingredients.[48] If you are intolerant of soy oil and soy lecithin, carefully check all of the oils you use as these ingredients are often included in margarine, oil blends, and cooking sprays.
- Soy is often present in products such as chocolate chips, frostings, dairy-free cheeses, mayonnaise, and confectionary sprinkles.
- Know which ingredients in the products you buy may be derived from soy. Words that often indicate the presence of soy are vegetable protein, textured vegetable protein or TVP®, plant protein, starch, vegetable broth, emulsifier, bulking agent, or stabilizer.[49] Check with the manufacturer if the source of any ingredient is not clearly identified to make sure it is not derived from soy.

The Art and Science of Gluten-free Baking

Baking with gluten-free flours is very different from baking with wheat flour. Because gluten is missing from flours such as millet, sorghum, and rice, the elasticity provided by the gluten protein in wheat flour is also missing. It is this elasticity that makes it possible for wheat-based dough to rise twice during the bread-making process, gives pizza crust its chewiness, and adds a lightness to cakes. The art of gluten-free baking involves mimicking the characteristics of wheat flour by using different types of flours and starches. For instance, in recipes requiring a little elasticity, bean flours are often used. The protein in bean flours such as fava and garbanzo flours makes it possible to roll out pie dough. Other flours such as millet can give baked goods a firm but light structure. Sweet rice flour gives baked goods a smoothness and light texture. Too much of any one flour, however, can ruin the taste of a recipe. For example, too much bean or quinoa flour can add a bitter taste. Carefully balancing the flours in a gluten-free baking mix is the key to the best tasting baked goods.

Some other pointers are needed as well:

1. Don't over-bake! As soon as a toothpick inserted in the baked good comes out without raw batter or wet crumbs attached, remove the baked good from the oven. Even a minute or two of over-baking will give you a dry product.

2. Use fresh baking powder only. Make sure your baking powder can has not been open for longer than two months. The combination of old baking powder and heavy gluten-free flours will prevent your baked goods from rising properly.

3. It will only rise once! Don't expect a gluten-free yeast dough to rise twice like wheat dough. Because gluten-free flours are heavy, they rise only once. Never punch down a ball of gluten-free dough after it has risen — it likely won't rise again.

4. Achieving lift. The heaviness of gluten-free flours makes sifting flour unnecessary. Lightness in gluten-free baked goods is achieved by using the correct combination of flours, baking soda, baking powder, and (for some recipes) yeast and some type of sugar. Adding acids that interact with baking soda and baking powder (e.g., apple cider vinegar and lemon juice) can also help the leavening process, and are especially recommended when using an egg replacer or a sugar substitute such as liquid stevia.

5. Measuring correctly. Obtaining the correct balance of dry and wet ingredients is essential in gluten-free baking. Use individual measuring cups (rather than a glass measuring cup marked with increments) for both dry and wet ingredients. Always measure flours by using a measuring cup that has been leveled off with the flat side of a knife. Be careful to add the correct amount of liquid as well; too much liquid will make your baked goods rise quickly and then shrivel upon cooling (using a non-dairy milk that is too high in water content could also cause this result). Measure shortening by packing it tightly into a measuring cup for accurate measurements. If a recipe calls for "melted shortening," measure it as a solid *before* melting it. Metric measurements are included for all recipes for those who prefer to weigh ingredients.

6. Freezing. Gluten-free baked goods taste best when served the day they are prepared. However, if you need to prepare items several days ahead of time, consider freezing them to maintain freshness. I freeze nearly everything ahead of time, including cakes, pies, pie dough, and cookies (do not freeze batter or frosted items). Pie dough freezes best when kneaded into a ball and wrapped tightly in freezer paper; to thaw, simply leave it at room temperature for two hours. To freeze a baked good, cool the item completely to room temperature after baking, cover with plastic wrap, seal in an airtight container, and place in the freezer. Thaw the uncovered and unwrapped baked good at room temperature for three hours; reheat briefly in the oven (5 to 10 minutes at 350° F) to bring back crispness. Avoid reheating custard and pumpkin pies, as the temperature extremes can cause them to crack and separate from the crust.

7. Enjoy the challenge! Experimenting with gluten-free flours can be an extremely healthful and rewarding experience. Gluten-free flours are much more nutritious than the processed, bleached wheat flour typically used for baking. They also have a richer flavor than wheat products which makes them as good to eat as to make.

Having a Gluten-free Kitchen

If you have Celiac Disease or are gluten sensitive, making sure that your cooking surfaces, utensils, pots, and pans, potholders, kitchen towels, and kitchen counters are free of gluten is essential. Even a crumb of a gluten-containing food could make someone who is highly sensitive to gluten ill. So how do you keep the gluten sensitive people in your home safe? Eliminating gluten entirely from the kitchen is the best way. Here are some suggestions for making this transition in your kitchen:

1. Keep it tasty! Going gluten-free doesn't mean that your food needs to be bland. No one will miss the gluten if the food is delicious. Using recipes that even the gluten-eaters in your house will enjoy makes the use of gluten in your kitchen unnecessary.

2. Clean out the kitchen. Carefully go through the food in your kitchen to remove items containing gluten. Give these items away to friends and family, or donate them to a food pantry. Scrub all cabinets, shelves, drawers, refrigerator and kitchen surfaces, and ovens to make sure all traces of gluten have been removed. Replace potholders, cloth kitchen towels, sponges, and cutting boards with new ones. Make sure old cookbooks are free of flour and crumbs as well.

3. Keep your cookware gluten-free. Cook only with pots and pans, bread machines, waffle irons, fryers, colanders, and other cookware that have not been previously used to make gluten-containing items. Never use your gluten-free cookware to make gluten-containing items.

4. When the guests arrive. Designate a place away from the kitchen where gluten-containing food gifts from guests can be placed, or, better yet, ask guests not to bring gluten-containing foods into your home. Since keeping gluten out of your kitchen is not always possible when guests visit, be sure to carefully wash all dishes, pots, pans, and other cookware just in case they have come in contact with gluten. If using a dishwasher, rinse your dishes before placing them into the dishwasher. Carefully wipe down all kitchen surfaces that may have come in contact with gluten. Use disposable paper towels in place of cloth towels for drying hands and counters.

5. Pet food. Feed pets and store pet food outside of the kitchen. "Grain free" pet foods may also be a good alternative, but check to make sure any products you choose are completely gluten free.

6. Store gluten separately. If you do store some gluten-containing foods in your home, find a storage area for them (preferably not in the kitchen) that is separate from where you store your gluten-free items.

7. Communicate with everyone in your household.
Getting all household members onboard with the new gluten-free status of the kitchen can be tricky! It is especially difficult for children to understand how certain foods can make the gluten sensitive members of the household sick. Talking to everyone openly about how they can help keep the kitchen safe is essential.

Storing Gluten-free Flours

Most gluten-free flours come in bags that generally range from 16 to 80 ounces (454 to 2268 g). Storing the flours in stackable containers (4 cups or 1 liter in size or larger) is needed. Label each container with the name of the flour it contains. Since the bags of gluten-free flour that you buy in the store are smaller than the typical bag of wheat flour, you may go through your flour supply quickly; store extra bags of each flour as back-up. For some flours (e.g., millet, sorghum, rice, and starches), storage in a cool, dark pantry is adequate. For other flours (nut meals, seed meals (e.g., flax meal), and bean flours), storage in the refrigerator is necessary to prevent the flour from spoiling. For those with a histamine intolerance, store bean flours and nut and seed meals in the freezer; remove them from the freezer one hour before use to thaw.

Adapting the Recipes for Other Dietary Needs

Although the recipes in this book are all gluten, dairy, and soy free (as long as the ingredients you use are), you may have additional food allergies, intolerances, or dietary limitations requiring additional changes to these recipes. Though it is not possible to include suggestions for all dietary concerns and intolerances, some suggestions for making recipe substitutions for some of the more common allergens are below. In addition, "Allergy/intolerance substitutions" and "Reduced sugar" suggestions are listed for each recipe. To make a substitution, continue to follow the steps identified in the original recipe, but replace or change the ingredients as specified in the "Allergy/intolerance substitutions" and "Reduced Sugar" sections of the recipe.

The information below and in the recipes is *not* intended to be a complete listing of all allergy-containing ingredients; always carefully check all of the ingredients you use to make sure they are safe for your health concerns. Contact the manufacturer if you are not sure if an ingredient contains an allergen or not. If you have a dietary concern that is not included below or if you are unsure about an ingredient, consult with your medical practitioner to identify a suitable replacement for the problem ingredient in the recipe. Most of all, thoroughly research your food intolerance or allergy to make sure you know all the sources of potential contamination for your food.

Corn Allergies

Corn is one of the most difficult allergens to avoid, simply because so many preservatives, sweeteners, colorings, flavorings, and additives are derived from corn. Corn is not identified as one of the eight major food allergens by the FDA, so manufacturers are not required to indicate the presence of corn on product labels. Cooking only with whole, unprocessed foods is the best way to avoid corn. While few of the recipes in this book include corn or corn syrup (except for the Corn Bread, Brownies, Old-fashioned Oatmeal Cookies, and All-but-the-kitchen-sink Bars), other ingredients (for example, xanthan gum, baking powder, brown sugar, yeast, vanilla extract, and confectioners' sugar) often either contain corn (usually as a starch or syrup) or are derived from corn. Some suggestions for avoiding corn include:

- Use brown rice syrup in place of corn syrup (be sure to check the syrup for additives such as caramel color that could be derived from corn).
- Use guar gum instead of xanthan gum in the gluten-free flour mix.
- Use a baking powder made with potato starch instead of corn starch.
- Avoid brands of brown sugar that contain caramel color.
- Avoid brands of yeast that are derived from corn.
- Check your vanilla extract to make sure that it is not made with corn syrup.
- Use a brand of confectioners' sugar made with a starch other than corn starch, or make your own at home (see page 70).

- Be sure to check all of the ingredients you use (in addition to the ones mentioned here) for potential corn contamination.

Egg-Related Concerns

Eggs are identified as one of the eight major food allergens by the FDA; manufacturers are thus required to indicate the presence of eggs on product labels. Most of the recipes in this book call for eggs, since eggs are very effective at binding ingredients together. For those following a vegan diet or who need to eliminate eggs from their diet for a health reason or allergy, egg substitutes or "replacers" are used. Recipes for homemade egg replacers (which tend to work better with gluten-free flours than most store-bought brands) are provided in the "Do-it-yourself Ingredient Recipes" section of this book (page 73). Other tips for eliminating eggs from recipes include:
- If you use a packaged egg replacer, make sure it does not contain egg, as some contain egg whites (albumen); follow the directions on the packaging before using it in the recipe.
- Products containing lecithin, emulsifiers, and preservatives (e.g., lysozyme) may also be derived from eggs[50]; contact the manufacturer if you are unsure about the source of any ingredient.

Histamine Intolerance

A histamine "intolerance" occurs when the body's level of histamine builds up, rather than being broken down naturally by histamine-degrading enzymes.[51] Although histamines are needed by the body for it to function correctly, in some individuals, too much histamine in the body can trigger a reaction similar to that of other food intolerances. Foods high in histamine, as well as those that trigger the body to release histamine, should be avoided by individuals with a histamine intolerance. These foods include (but are not limited to) canned, smoked, or fermented foods (e.g., canned tuna, soy sauce, wine, yogurt, yeast breads, some vinegars), egg whites, strawberries, citrus fruits, bananas, pineapple, papaya, spinach, avocado, tomato, algae (e.g., carrageenan, agar, seaweed), certain spices (e.g., black and white pepper, cayenne, hot paprika, cinnamon, ginger, cumin, cloves, nutmeg), vanilla, cocoa, chocolate, carob, flours containing gluten, buckwheat, soy, many preservatives and food dyes, many nuts and seeds (e.g., pecans and flax), some dried fruits, collagen and gelatin, and aged cheeses or meats.[52, 53] Products containing alcohol (e.g., liquors, flavored extracts) and caffeinated teas may also be harmful to individuals with a histamine intolerance as they are thought to interfere with the production of diamine oxidase (DAO), an enzyme that breaks down histamine in the digestive tract.[54]

Individuals with a histamine intolerance often react differently to different foods, making it necessary to know which foods trigger a reaction in each individual. **Because of the difficulty in adapting each recipe to an individual's specific histamine triggers, suggestions for reducing histamine are *not* provided for each recipe**. Know which foods trigger a reaction for you before making any recipe. Some basic substitutions to consider are:
- Individuals who are sensitive to the histamine in egg whites may wish to use only egg yolks (use two egg yolks to replace one whole egg or egg white) or an egg-free substitute; it is important to note that

some medical practitioners recommend avoiding eggs completely.[55]
- Follow the "reduced sugar" instructions for the recipes in this book if recommended by your medical practitioner.
- Avoid recipes that include ingredients such as bananas, strawberries, raspberries, cocoa, citrus, chocolate chips, yeast, yogurt, and probiotics. Some individuals may also be sensitive to foods such as pumpkin, dried fruits, peppers, garlic, and onions; avoid recipes containing these ingredients or leave the ingredient out if needed.
- Leave out vinegars (e.g., apple cider vinegar) and spices (e.g., cinnamon, ginger, nutmeg, cloves, cayenne) if sensitive to them. If you tolerate white distilled vinegar, use it as a replacement for apple cider vinegar.
- Leave out nuts and seeds such as pecans, sunflower seeds, and flax. Although almonds are generally tolerated by individuals with a histamine intolerance[56], substitutions for almond-based ingredients are given in the "Allergy/Intolerance Substitutions: Tree nuts" section of each recipe for those who are sensitive to them. Cashews may also be tolerated by some individuals; avoid recipes containing cashews if needed.
- Replace flavored abstracts (e.g., vanilla) with an equivalent measure of maple syrup.
- For the pie dough recipes, use water in place of wine or vodka.
- Replace flax meal and bean flour with quinoa flour if tolerated.
- Replace the bean flour in the Rising and Non-rising Egg Replacer recipes with quinoa flour if tolerated.

- Do not use the Flax Meal Egg Replacer. Use the Chia Seed Egg Replacer only if chia seeds are tolerated.
- Leave out the gelatin if it is not tolerated; if it is tolerated, use only plain, unflavored gelatin. Gelatin can also be replaced with agar powder if tolerated.
- Avoid using sunflower, walnut, or soy oils; olive oil, coconut oil, palm oil shortening, and lard (preservative free and organic only) are generally tolerated.
- For the Poultry Stuffing recipe, avoid using store-bought sausage (make your own sausage using only herbs and spices that are tolerated). If the collagen in chicken broth is not tolerated, use a homemade vegetable broth.

It is important to note that the suggestions above are aimed at reducing the intake of histamine rather than eliminating it, and so might not be suitable for highly sensitive individuals. Please consult a medical practitioner for additional recipe adaptations needed for your specific health conditions. A regularly-updated list of histamine compatible foods is available online through the Swiss Interest Group Histamine Intolerance at "www.histamintoleranz.ch". The foods discussed above for removal from recipes were identified from this list as "incompatible" or "very poorly tolerated" at the time of the printing of this book; changes may occur to this list as updates become available.

Nightshade (Tomato) Family Sensitivities

Nightshade plants include tomatoes, potatoes, eggplants, and peppers, as well as common nightshade (*Solanum nigrum*), a toxic plant for which the family is named. The nightshade family does *not* include the spice, black pepper. The alkaloids contained in many of the Nightshades are known to increase inflammation in the body, worsening arthritis in some individuals[57] and possibly affecting intestinal inflammation as well. Allergies and sensitivities to tomatoes in particular exist. If you are sensitive to plants in the Nightshade family, use either arrowroot or tapioca starch in place of potato starch in the gluten-free flour mix recipe; avoid using tomato sauce with the Pizza Dough recipe; do not include green chilies or the hot pepper sauce in the Corn Bread recipe; and leave out the cayenne pepper in the Carrot Spice Bread, Honey & Spice Cookie, and Gingerbread Cookie recipes.

Oil Sensitivities

For those with specific allergies or intolerances to oils (such as canola or soy), check the ingredients on your cooking oil, shortening, and cooking spray to make sure they do not contain the oil to which you are sensitive. Some individuals with a soy intolerance may tolerate soy lecithin; know what you tolerate prior to using any product that contains soy lecithin (e.g., store-bought cooking sprays). The simplest solution to avoiding undesired oils in a cooking spray is to purchase an oil sprayer from a kitchen supply store and fill it with pure olive oil or another neutral-flavored oil that you tolerate. If you have a sensitivity to soy or canola oil, GF vegan palm-oil-based shortenings (e.g., Spectrum®) work well with the recipes in this book. Make sure the palm oil you purchase is organic, ethically sourced, and without additives. For those with a salicylate intolerance, please consult a medical practitioner when choosing any oils or shortenings as some (e.g., olive, palm, and coconut oils) are high in salicylates; preservative-free, organic lard is an alternative for those with a salicylate intolerance.

Peanut Allergies

Peanuts are identified as one of the eight major allergens by the FDA, and thus are supposed to be listed on food labels if present in a product. Although none of the recipes in this book include peanuts, when baking for someone with a peanut allergy, it is essential that all ingredients be carefully screened for potential peanut contamination. Many brands of packaged nuts, candies, other packaged foods, and vegetable oils contain peanut proteins and oils. Read all packaging carefully to make sure that peanuts are not listed as an ingredient and that trace amounts of peanuts have not been added during processing or packaging. If the packaging does not clearly specify if peanuts are present, contact the manufacturer directly to find out. Some people who have peanut allergies may be allergic to other nuts as well; be sure to find out if the person for whom you are baking has other allergies.

Rice Allergies

Although rare, rice allergies and intolerances do occur in some individuals. If sensitive to rice, make sure that the ingredients you use do not include rice flour, traces of rice resulting from the manufacturing process, or other ingredients derived from rice. When making a substitution for brown rice flour, leave out the rice flour and add an equivalent amount of any other gluten-free flour that is tolerated (e.g., amaranth); if replacing sweet rice flour, use a starch (e.g., tapioca) instead. Specific suggestions for replacing rice flour are included throughout this book and in Table 1 (page 68).

Salicylate Intolerance

Salicylates are a type of chemical found naturally in many fruits, herbs, and vegetables; they also come in synthetic forms that are used in the manufacture of many medicines and other products (e.g., the salicylic acid found in aspirin). Reactions to the amount of salicylates found in different foods vary greatly between individuals. Some ingredients used in this book that are usually not tolerated by those with a salicylate intolerance include almonds, blueberries, blackberries, raspberries, strawberries, most varieties of apples, peaches, dried fruits, corn syrup, cornmeal, olive oil, coconut oil, palm oil, coconut, coconut milk, hot peppers, zucchini, carrots, most herbs and spices, many seeds (including chia, flax, and pumpkin), citrus fruits, molasses, honey, yeast, tomato sauce, fava/broad beans (often used to make bean flour), wine and many other types of alcohol (plain, unflavored vodka is an exception since it usually contains a negligible amount of salicylates), and many preservatives, flavored extracts, and food colorings. [58, 59, 60, 61] Because salicylates are often concentrated in the skins of fruits and vegetables, both Golden Delicious apples and pears (two fruits low in salicylates) should be peeled before adding them to any recipe. Use Golden Delicious apples only as other varieties of apple contain higher levels of salicylates.

The recipes in this book should not be used by those who are highly sensitive or allergic to salicylates. In addition, because of the extensive list of foods not tolerated by those with a salicylate intolerance and the variation in how individuals react to foods containing salicylates, substitution suggestions for this intolerance are *not* included for each recipe in this book.

Some basic substitutions to consider to reduce (but not completely eliminate) the amount of salicylates in recipes are:

- Avoid recipes containing almonds, corn meal, corn flour, fresh corn, all types of berries, zucchini, carrot, pumpkin, yeast, citrus, coconut, coconut butter, and coconut milk, unless a safe substitution for the problem ingredient can be made.
- Replace olive, palm, corn, and coconut oils with oils that are tolerated (e.g., safflower and sunflower seed oils are usually tolerated). Similarly, replace vegetable-based shortenings with either preservative-free, organic lard or, if dairy is tolerated, butter.
- If potato starch is not tolerated, replace it with arrowroot starch or tapioca starch (though some individuals may not tolerate these either).
- Leave out hot pepper sauces, chilies, and jalapenos.
- Avoid using fava (broad) bean flour; garbanzo bean flour is low in salicylates and generally tolerated.
- Replace berries and peaches with fruits that are low in salicylates (e.g., bananas, peeled pears, peeled Golden Delicious apples).
- When adding chopped or sliced apples to a recipe, use only peeled Golden Delicious apples (if

tolerated). Replace store-bought applesauce with fresh homemade applesauce made from peeled Golden Delicious apples.
- Replace almond meal with sunflower seed, cashew, or hazelnut meal if tolerated (follow the recipe for seed and nut meals in the "Do-it-yourself Ingredients" section). These nuts and seeds contain low levels of salicylates which may not be suitable for everyone.
- Sweeteners: Replace honey with pure maple syrup or additive-free rice syrup. Leave out molasses. Use additive-free rice syrup in place of corn syrup. White cane sugar and additive-free brown sugar contain negligible amounts of salicylates and can be kept in recipes. It is unclear if stevia is safe for those with a salicylate intolerance; avoid if needed.
- Leave out dried fruits (e.g., raisins, dried cranberries).
- Use preservative-free rice milk as the "milk of choice" (see the recipe for making it yourself in the "Do-it-yourself Ingredients" section).
- Leave out vinegars, spices (e.g., cinnamon, nutmeg, cloves, ginger, cayenne), seeds, flavored extracts, and citrus zest and juice. Extracts can be replaced with an equivalent amount of pure maple syrup.
- Use GF unflavored vodka (if tolerated) or water in place of wine in the pie dough recipes.
- Check the ingredient labels of chocolate chips to make sure they are not made from high-salicylate oils (e.g., palm).
- Replace flax meal with quinoa flour or amaranth flour, if tolerated.
- Use eggs as indicated in the recipes, or replace them with the Rising and Non-rising Egg Replacers

(pages 74 to 76; follow the "salicylate" substitution suggestions for the egg replacer recipes). Do not use the flax meal or chia seed egg replacers as both are high in salicylates.
- For the poultry stuffing recipe, make your own pork sausage and chicken broth using spices that you tolerate; leave out the herbs.

Several food guides for salicylate sensitivity can be found online and are listed in the reference section of this book. The foods identified in the list above were identified from these lists as containing low to negligible amounts of salicylates, which might not be adequate for highly sensitive individuals. Please consult a medical practitioner to make sure that all ingredients used for these recipes take into account the foods that trigger your salicylate intolerance.

Sugar Concerns

Sugars are found in many ingredients — not just cane sugar. Honey, maple syrup, molasses, corn syrup, rice syrup, nuts, and both dried and fresh fruits (e.g., raisins, blueberries, apples, apple sauce, apple cider vinegar, bananas) contain natural sugars such as glucose and fructose.[62] Sugars may also be found in other ingredients such as non-dairy and dairy milks, and some flours such as teff and millet.

Because of the difficulty in adapting any recipe to sugar-related health conditions such as diabetes or fructose sensitivity, specific substitutions are not provided for these conditions. Please consult a certified nutritionist or

medical practitioner if you wish to adapt the recipes in this book to these or other sugar-related health concerns.

For those interested in cutting back on their sugar in-take, "reduced sugar" instructions are included for many recipes in this book. Although most of these instructions call for clear, alcohol-free liquid stevia in place of sugar, some recipes also include unsweetened applesauce (which contains fructose) as a flavor enhancer. The main differences you will see between the reduced sugar and original recipes are that cakes and breads will not rise or brown quite as well without the sugar. In addition, because sugar gives structure to baked goods, the addition of other ingredients is often needed to prevent cakes and breads from collapsing as they cool; directions for adding these extra ingredients are given as needed in the "reduced sugar" directions. Because sugars such as cane sugar and honey boost the flavor of baked goods, the "reduced sugar" recipes will seem a little bland to those unused to a low sugar diet. Finally, check with your medical practitioner before using stevia to make sure it is suitable for your health conditions.

Tree Nut and Coconut Allergies

Tree nuts, coconut, and almond extract are ingredients in many of the recipes in this book. The U.S. Food and Drug Administration categorizes coconuts as tree nuts[63], even though coconuts are seeds produced by trees in the palm family and unrelated to tree nut species such as almond, cashew, and pecan. If a recipe is heavily based on coconut and no substitution is provided (e.g., the Chocolate Coconut Ganache recipe), those with a coconut allergy or intolerance should avoid the recipe completely.

Substitutions for coconut are listed separately from those for tree nuts in the "Allergy/Intolerance Substitutions" section of each recipe.

For those with a tree nut allergy or intolerance, you will need to make substitutions for the pecans, cashews, and almonds used in the recipes in this book. Replace pecans, cashews, and almonds with sunflower or pumpkin seeds (if tolerated) or leave out the nuts completely. Replace the almond extract in recipes with a different gluten-free extract (e.g., vanilla) or with pure maple syrup. Almond meal can be replaced with a different high-protein flour such as garbanzo or fava bean flour, pumpkin or sunflower seed meal, or quinoa flour. Avoid the Cashew-coconut Cream Topping and Moist Almond Crumb Cake recipes. Be sure to verify that all ingredients (including flours and starches) have not been processed in manufacturing plants that process tree nuts and/or coconut.

Flour Substitutions

Depending on your food allergies, intolerances, or other dietary needs, you may need to make substitutions in the flours and/or starches you use when baking. When making substitutions to either the gluten-free flour mix recipe or the other recipes in this book, use flours that are similar to the ones being removed. Table 1 (page 68) identifies some possible substitutions, but you will need to try different flours to see which you prefer.

You may notice some slight differences in baked goods made with the substitutes (e.g., the recipes may not rise as well, or may have a slightly different flavor or texture). The trick is to not use too much of any one flour when making a substitution. If a recipe already includes a specific flour, do not add more of it when making a substitution; choose a different flour instead. Little change in the final baked good will be noticed when making substitutions for starches, as long as another starch is used.

Some flours have specific characteristics that need to be considered before use. Flours with particularly strong flavors are bean (slightly bitter taste), quinoa (slightly bitter taste), teff (slight mineral taste and dark color), and buckwheat (slight mineral taste and dark color); avoid adding more than ¼ cup (about 32 grams) of any of these flours to a recipe, unless otherwise directed in the recipe. Only small amounts (1 to 2 Tablespoons, or 4.5 to 9 grams) of coconut flour should be added to any recipe as this flour tends to absorb liquid and will make the batter dry (for this reason, coconut flour has been excluded from Table 1). Some flours contain natural sugars (e.g., millet and teff flours) and may be a concern for those with sugar-related health problems. Other flours may be a problem for those with a histamine intolerance (e.g., buckwheat) or salicylate intolerance (e.g., almond meal and corn meal). Non-organic flours may also be a problem for those with sensitive digestive systems as some may contain glyphosate, an ingredient in herbicides sometimes used before harvest on grains such as sorghum and corn. It is thought that glyphosate harms the digestive system by causing imbalances in the bacteria in the gut, triggering various health conditions.[64] To reduce glyphosate in your diet, use organic flours if possible. Finally, some flours may contain naturally-occurring chemicals that you may wish to avoid (e.g., trace amounts of arsenic in brown rice flour). Be sure to consult a medical practitioner about the flours or starches discussed in this book prior to use.

Table 1. Possible flour and starch substitutes.

Type & texture of flour	Flour included in recipe	Suitable flour & starch substitutions
• Whole grain, ground • High fiber and protein • Fine texture • Gives structure to finished product	Sorghum	Teff; Buckwheat; Amaranth; Quinoa; Corn flour (not meal or starch); Millet
	Millet	Teff; Buckwheat; Amaranth; Quinoa; Corn flour (not meal or starch); Sorghum
	Corn flour (not meal or starch)	Teff; Buckwheat; Amaranth; Quinoa; Sorghum; Millet
• Whole grain, ground • High fiber and protein • Moderate texture • Makes dough flexible	Fava or garbanzo bean flour	Quinoa; Amaranth
• Whole grain, ground • High fiber and protein • Moderate to dense texture • Good for moisture retention	Almond meal	Pumpkin or sunflower seed meal; Certified GF oat flour; Dry quinoa flakes
	Certified GF oat flour	Dry quinoa flakes; Almond or other nut meal; Pumpkin or Sunflower seed meal; Flax meal

Type & texture of flour	Flour included in recipe	Suitable flour & starch substitutions
- **Whole grain, ground** - **High fiber and protein** - **Gritty texture** - **Adds structure and/or crispness to recipes**	Brown rice	Corn flour (not meal or starch); Teff; Quinoa; Buckwheat; Amaranth; Bean flour
	Corn meal	Brown rice flour; Flax meal; Chia seed meal; Certified GF oat flour
	Certified GF rolled oats	Dry quinoa flakes; Flax meal; Brown rice flour;
	Flax meal	Chia seed meal; Certified GF oat flour
- **High starch content** - **Fine texture** - **Makes recipes light**	Potato starch	Arrowroot starch; Tapioca starch; Sweet rice flour; Corn starch
	Sweet rice flour	Arrowroot starch; Tapioca starch; Corn starch; Potato starch
	Arrowroot starch	Tapioca starch; Sweet rice flour; Corn starch; Potato starch
	Tapioca starch	Arrowroot starch; Sweet rice flour; Corn starch; Potato starch

Do-It-Yourself Ingredient Recipes

For those who wish to avoid preservatives or specific allergens, making your own ingredients can be an inexpensive and healthy option. Some simple recipes are below. Most take about ten minutes to prepare.

Confectioners' Sugar

Place 1 cup (200 g) pure super-fine cane sugar in a food processor; add ¼ cup (30 g) tapioca starch or arrowroot starch. Process for about 5 minutes till the texture of the sugar mixture feels smooth when rubbed between your fingers (note: cover the food processor with a towel while processing to prevent fine sugar particles from escaping into the air). Store in a sealed container at room temperature. Homemade confectioners' sugar is usually not as finely ground as the store-bought kind, but works fairly well in most recipes.

Coconut Milk

☑ **Allergy/Intolerance Substitutions:**
Coconut: Avoid this recipe.
Salicylate: Avoid this recipe.

Use either fresh coconut meat (brown peel removed and food processed till finely shredded) or dehydrated, unsweetened, shredded organic coconut. Place ½ cup (35 g) of the shredded coconut in a heavy-duty blender (do not use a food processor). Pour in 2 cups (473 ml) of warm filtered or spring water (100 – 110° F or 38 – 43° C; using hotter water will release a higher proportion of coconut oil into the coconut milk which may not be desired). If you are using dehydrated coconut, let the coconut soak for one hour in the water to re-hydrate; if fresh coconut is being used, you do not need to soak the coconut. Blend the coconut and water mixture for one to two minutes till the liquid is creamy in color. Place a large, fine mesh sieve on top of a bowl. Pour the liquid into the sieve, pushing the liquid through the sieve with a rubber spatula till only the dry fibers of the coconut remain (you may need to clean the coconut fibers out of the sieve once to get the liquid through). Store any unused milk in a sealed glass container in the refrigerator for up to one week. Shake the milk prior to use. Unlike many canned coconut milks, homemade coconut milk is free of preservatives and thickeners, but will be too thin to use in recipes specifically requiring coconut cream (e.g., frosting); use canned, preservative-free coconut milk for these recipes instead.

Nut Milk

☑ Allergy/Intolerance Substitutions:
Tree nuts: Avoid this recipe.
Histamine: Use only almonds (if tolerated); otherwise, avoid this recipe.
Salicylate: If you tolerate a low level of salicylates, use cashews or hazelnuts; otherwise, avoid this recipe.

Place ½ cup (80 g) of raw GF nuts (e.g., almonds, cashews, hazelnuts) in a heavy-duty blender (do not use a food processor); pour in 2 cups (473 ml) of cool water, and blend for one to two minutes till the liquid is creamy in color. Place a fine mesh sieve on top of a bowl. Pour the liquid into the sieve, pushing the liquid through the sieve with a rubber spatula (reserve the nut meal that remains in the sieve for other recipes). You can stop at this point in this recipe for nut milk that will be used for baking; for nut milk that you plan to drink, pour the sieved milk through two layers of cheese cloth to remove any remaining small pieces of nut. Store unused milk in a sealed glass container in the refrigerator for up to one week. Shake prior to use.

Rice Milk

☑ **Allergy/Intolerance Substitutions:**
Rice: Avoid this recipe.

Place ⅔ cup (120 g) of cooked and cooled white or brown rice in a heavy-duty blender (do not use a food processor). Pour in 2 cups (473 ml) of cool, filtered or spring water, and blend for one to two minutes till the liquid is creamy in color. Place a large, fine mesh sieve on top of a bowl. Pour the liquid into the sieve, pushing the liquid through the sieve with a rubber spatula (clean the rice hull pieces out of the sieve as needed to get the liquid through). Store unused milk in a sealed glass container in the refrigerator for up to one week. Shake the milk prior to use.

Pumpkin Seed or Sunflower Seed Meal

☑ **Allergy/Intolerance Substitutions:**
Histamine: Avoid this recipe.
Salicylate: If you tolerate a low level of salicylates, use sunflower seeds (avoid pumpkin seeds).

Place 1¼ cup (160 g) of sunflower or pumpkin seeds (with shells removed) in a food processor. Process until a fine meal is obtained. This recipe makes approximately 1 cup (160 g) of seed meal. Store the seed meal in the refrigerator or freezer.

Egg Replacers

Egg replacers or substitutes are easy to make at home. Use the Rising Egg Replacer in cakes, breads, and other baked goods that need to rise; the Non-rising Egg Replacer in cookies and pie dough; and the Flax Meal and Chia Seed Egg Replacers in granola and heavy breads. Because the Rising and Non-rising Egg Replacer recipes have been specially created for this book, they tend to work better than store-bought egg replacers for these recipes.

The amount of egg replacer to use for each recipe is identified throughout this book. In general, ¼ cup (59 ml) of egg substitute (provided by each of the egg replacer recipes below) equals about one large egg. Recipes containing egg replacers may require a longer baking time than needed for the original recipes. These egg replacers should not be used as a substitute for the egg whites in meringue, as an egg substitute in quiche or omelets, or as an egg wash for brushing the tops of scones or pie dough prior to baking (skip the egg wash step entirely if needed).

1. Flax Meal Egg Replacer
Use in hearty breads, muffins, and granola.

☑ **Allergy/Intolerance Substitutions:**
Histamine: Avoid this recipe.
Salicylate: Avoid this recipe.

Directions:
Living Without's: Gluten-free & More magazine provides an easy flax meal egg replacer recipe. Whisk 1 T. (6.5 g) flax meal with 3 T. (45 ml) hot tap water. Let the mixture thicken for 10 minutes, stirring occasionally.[65]

2. Chia Seed Egg Replacer
Use in hearty breads, muffins, and granola.

☑ Allergy/Intolerance Substitutions:
<u>Histamine:</u> Avoid if you do not tolerate chia seeds.
<u>Salicylate:</u> Avoid this recipe.

Directions:
Whisk together for one minute 2 t. (6 g) of chia seed with 3 T. plus 1 t. (50 ml) hot tap water. Let the mixture thicken for 10 minutes, stirring occasionally, before adding to your recipe. Though chia seed often works better as an egg replacer than flax meal, the small seeds can make baked goods look spotted and may add an unwanted crunch.

3. Rising Egg Replacer
Use for baked goods that need to rise (i.e., cakes, breads, scones, and pizza dough).

☑ Allergy/Intolerance Substitutions:
<u>Bovine/Porcine:</u> Use agar powder instead of gelatin.
<u>Histamine:</u> If tolerated: use quinoa flour instead of bean flour; use agar powder instead of gelatin or leave out; and replace the apple cider vinegar with distilled white vinegar or leave out.
<u>Salicylate:</u> If tolerated, use garbanzo bean flour and unflavored, powdered gelatin (fava/broad bean flour and agar powder are high in salicylates, as are many flavored gelatins). Leave out the apple cider vinegar.

Ingredients:
⅓ c. bean flour (garbanzo or fava) or quinoa flour (40 g)
¼ c. arrowroot starch (30 g)
⅓ c. tapioca starch (44 g)
1 T. baking powder (15 g)
1 t. baking soda (5 g)
1½ t. unflavored gelatin powder or agar powder (4.5 g)
1 t. apple cider vinegar (5 ml)

Directions:
Step 1. Mix together the dry ingredients in a 2-cup (½-liter) storage container. Store the sealed container at room temperature till use. Shake to recombine the ingredients prior to use.

Step 2. For the equivalent of one egg, whisk together in a small bowl the egg replacer powder and water as follows:

For recipes labeled specifically as "cakes":
1 T. (6 g) egg replacer powder with 3 T. (45 ml) water.

For other recipes requiring the "Rising Egg Replacer":
2 T. (12 g) egg replacer powder with 2 T. (30 ml) water.

Step 3. Let the mixture rest at room temperature for 5 minutes; whisk again.

Step 4. Whisk in 1 t. (5 ml) apple cider vinegar per "egg," and immediately add the egg replacer to the batter. (Note: this egg replacer loses its "lift" if allowed to rest on the counter after adding the vinegar; bake as directed in the recipe as soon as the batter is mixed.)

4. Non-rising Egg Replacer
Use for cookies and doughs that do not need to rise.

☑ **Allergy/Intolerance Substitutions:**
Bovine/Porcine: Use agar powder instead of gelatin.
Histamine: If tolerated: use quinoa flour instead of bean flour; use agar powder instead of gelatin or leave out.
Salicylate: If tolerated, use garbanzo bean flour and unflavored, powdered gelatin (fava/broad bean flour and agar powder are high in salicylates, as are many flavored gelatins).

Ingredients:
⅓ c. bean flour (garbanzo or fava) or quinoa flour (40 g)
¼ c. arrowroot starch (30 g)
⅓ c. tapioca starch (44 g)
1½ t. unflavored gelatin powder or agar powder (4.5 g)

Directions:
Step 1. Mix together the ingredients in a 2-cup (½-liter) storage container. Store the container sealed at room temperature till use. Shake to recombine the ingredients prior to use.

Step 2. For the equivalent of one egg, whisk in a small bowl 2 T. (12 g) of the egg replacer powder with 2 T. (30 ml) of water. Let the mixture rest at room temperature for 5 minutes.

Step 3. Whisk prior to adding to your recipe. (Note: do not add apple cider vinegar as specified in the Rising Egg Replacer recipe.)

Easy Breakfast Recipes

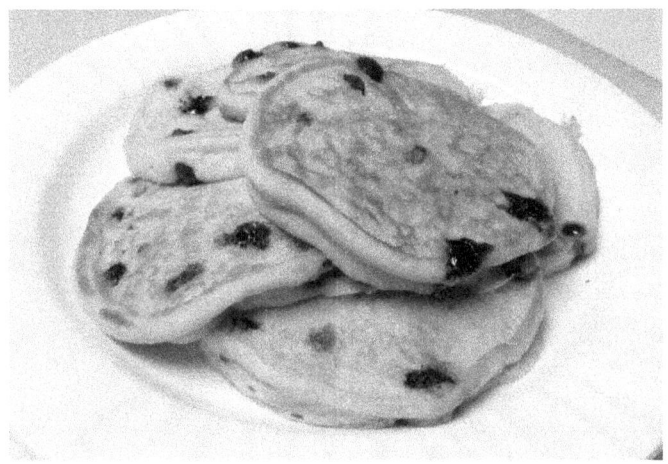

Granola

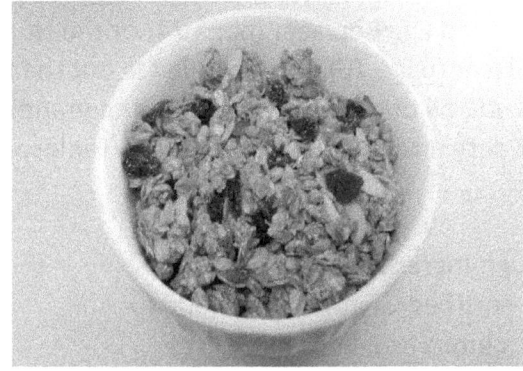

A nutritious breakfast cereal is actually very easy to make and costs much less than the packaged allergen-free cereals (it tastes better, too). If you like and tolerate coconut, add ½ cup (35 g) of shredded, unsweetened coconut to the dry ingredients in step 1. Serve the granola with a non-dairy milk, or sprinkle the granola on fresh Coconut Yogurt (see page 261). Makes approximately 8 cups (880 g).

☑ **Allergy/Intolerance Substitutions:**

Tree nuts: In step 1, leave out the almond meal or replace it with flax meal, sunflower seed meal, pumpkin seed meal, or shredded, unsweetened coconut (if tolerated). In step 7, leave out the sliced almonds, or replace with raw pumpkin seeds or sunflower seeds.

Eggs: Prepare the equivalent of two whole eggs using the Chia Seed Egg Replacer (page 74) or the Non-rising Egg Replacer (page 76). In step 2, leave out the egg whites and add all of the egg replacer.

Oats: Avoid this recipe.

☑ Reduced Sugar:

In step 2, leave out the honey; add 80 drops of clear, alcohol-free liquid stevia, an extra ¼ cup (59 ml) oil (i.e., ½ cup or 118 ml oil total), an extra ½ t. (1.5 g) cinnamon (i.e., 2 t. or 6 g cinnamon total), and 1 extra whole egg (i.e., in addition to the two egg whites). If using an egg substitute, prepare the equivalent of 3 whole eggs using either the Chia Seed Egg Replacer (page 74) or the Non-rising Egg Replacer (page 76). In step 2, leave out the two egg whites and add all of the egg replacer. If the granola appears powdery after mixing, add an extra Tablespoon (15 ml) of oil.

Dough Ingredients:
5 c. certified GF rolled oats (500 g)
¾ c. gluten-free flour mix (96 g)
¼ c. almond meal (25 g)
1½ t. cinnamon (4.5 g)
⅔ c. honey (248 g)
2 egg whites
¼ c. pure olive oil (not extra virgin) or other neutral-flavored oil (59 ml)
½ c. sliced almonds (optional) (50 g)

Preheat Oven: 325° F/163° C

Directions:

Step 1. In a large mixing bowl, mix the oats, gluten-free flour mix, almond meal, and cinnamon with a rubber spatula till well combined.

Step 2. In a small mixing bowl, whisk together the honey, egg whites, and oil. Add to the oat/flour mixture; combine thoroughly till all of the oats are well-coated with the honey mixture, and all of the flour is mixed in.

Step 3. Pour the granola mixture into an 11" x 15" (28 cm x 38 cm) baking pan, leaving clumps of granola as you gently spread it out in the pan. Bake for 12 minutes.

Step 4. Gently flip the granola over in the pan with a metal spatula, being careful not to break up the oat clusters. Pull the granola away from the edges of the pan and into the center of the pan to prevent it from burning around the edges. Spread the granola out in the pan again, and place it back into the oven. Bake for another 6 minutes.

Step 5. Gently flip the granola over with a metal spatula, pulling the granola away from the edges of the pan and then spreading it out in the pan. Bake for another 6 minutes.

Step 6. Repeat Step 5.

Step 7. Sprinkle the sliced almonds on top of the granola. Bake another 5 to 8 minutes till all of the granola clusters are golden brown (or bake 5 to 8 minutes without the almonds).

Step 8. Remove the pan from the oven and cool the granola completely.

Step 9. Mix in any additional dried or roasted ingredients you wish (e.g., dried cranberries, raisins, shelled sunflower seeds, flax seeds, other nuts, etc.).

Step 10. Store at room temperature in an air-tight container for up to one week. Store in the refrigerator to keep it longer.

Nutritional content: Makes 16 servings (½ cup (67 g) per serving; includes sliced almonds). Each serving contains: Calories (250); Total Fat (8 g); Saturated Fat (1 g); Cholesterol (0 mg); Sodium (50 mg); Potassium (45 mg); Total Carbohydrate (38 g); Dietary Fiber (4 g); Sugars (11 g); Protein (7 g). Nutrient(s) of note (percent of Daily Value): Calcium 2%, Iron 10%

Pancakes

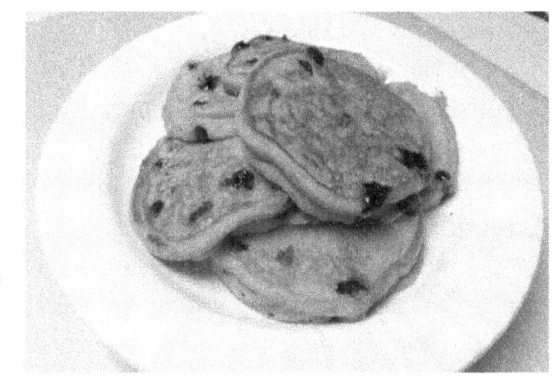

This recipe makes light and fluffy pancakes -- the kind you thought you'd never taste again after going gluten-free. The recipe below makes about six four-inch (10-cm) diameter pancakes (enough for one hungry person or three light eaters).

☑ Allergy/Intolerance Substitutions:
Eggs: Prepare the equivalent of one egg using the Rising Egg Replacer (page 74) or flax meal egg replacer (page 73). Leave out the egg in step 2, and add the egg replacer (if using the Rising Egg Replacer, be sure to add the apple cider vinegar as specified in the egg replacer recipe).

☑ Reduced Sugar:
In step 1, leave out the sugar. In step 2, add 6 to 10 drops of clear, alcohol-free liquid stevia.

Batter Ingredients:
1 c. gluten-free flour mix (130 g)
1 t. baking powder (5 g)
1 T. refined cane sugar (optional) (13 g)
1 large egg
1 T. pure olive oil (not extra virgin) or other neutral-flavored oil (15 ml)
1 c. hot tap water (237 ml)
¼ c. fresh blueberries (washed and dried), or peeled and chopped apple (optional) (35 g)

Directions:
Step 1. Mix together the dry ingredients.

Step 2. Add the egg, oil, and hot water. Mix together with a rubber spatula for one minute to form a smooth batter that is the consistency of thick cake batter; scrape the sides of the bowl as you mix.

Step 3. Let the batter rest at room temperature for 10 minutes to activate the baking powder.

Step 4. While the batter is resting, place the griddle or frying pan on a burner (or burners, if using a long griddle) set to medium. Let the griddle get hot.

Step 5. After the batter has rested, gently fold in the blueberries or small chunks of peeled apple if desired (make sure to blot the blueberries dry before adding them if they are wet).

Step 6. Spray the hot griddle with cooking spray. Ladle approximately ¼-cup (66 g) of the batter onto the griddle. Using the bottom of the ladle, gently spread the batter out to form a pancake that is approximately 4 inches (10 cm) in diameter and ½-inch (about 1 cm) thick; repeat for the other pancakes.

Step 7. When the bottom of the pancake is golden brown and the edges of the pancake start to look slightly dry, flip the pancake and cook the other side till it is golden brown. Don't overcook the pancakes (they will look slightly wrinkled if you do). Remove promptly from the griddle and enjoy!

Nutritional content: Makes 3 servings (2 pancakes (168 g) per serving, blueberries included). Each serving contains: Calories (260); Total Fat (7 g); Saturated Fat (1 g); Cholesterol (60 mg); Sodium (450 mg); Potassium (67 mg); Total Carbohydrate (46 g); Dietary Fiber (2 g); Sugars (6 g); Protein (4 g). Nutrient(s) of note (percent of Daily Value): Vitamin A 2%, Calcium 8%, Vitamin C 2%, Iron 10%

Batter-Dipped Fried Food and Fritters:

This pancake batter recipe makes a delicious batter for deep-frying foods. Pour 2 quarts (1.9 liters) of oil into a sauce pan and heat to 350° F (177° C). (Note: be sure to use an oil that has a smoke point above 400° F or 204° C.) In step 1, leave out the baking powder. In step 2, add an extra 2 Tablespoons (30 ml) of water to the 1 cup (237 ml) of hot tap water already included. After mixing the batter, dip in a bite-sized (or larger) chunk of seafood, fruit, or vegetable till it is completely coated with the batter. Let any excess batter drip off. Using a long-handled fork, carefully place the batter-dipped chunk in the heated oil (use caution in case the oil splatters). Repeat for 5 to 6 other pieces. Stir the chunks in the oil with a slotted spoon to prevent them from sticking together. When the bottom of each has turned golden brown, flip it over to cook the other side. When that side is golden brown, remove from the oil and drain on a paper-towel-lined platter. Let the oil return to 350° F/177° C before frying other pieces.

Waffles

These waffles turn out crispy on the outside and light on the inside. The batter is similar to that used for the pancakes with just a few modifications. Serve with fresh fruit and a little Coconut Yogurt (page 261), or with maple syrup. Makes 2 large waffles.

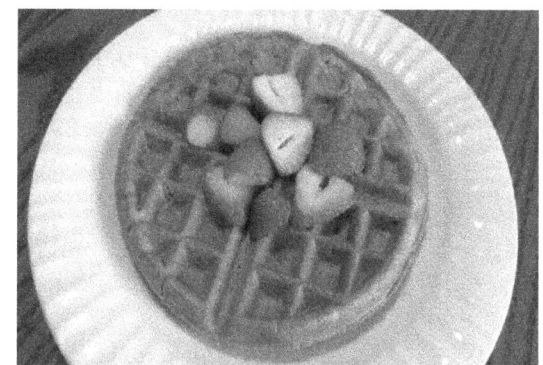

☑ Allergy/Intolerance Substitutions:
Eggs: Prepare the equivalent of one egg using the Rising Egg Replacer (page 74) or flax meal egg replacer (page 73). Leave out the egg in step 2, and add the egg replacer. If using the Rising Egg Replacer, be sure to add the apple cider vinegar as specified in the egg replacer recipe.

☑ Reduced Sugar:
In step 1, leave out the sugar. In step 2, add 6 to 10 drops of clear, alcohol-free liquid stevia.

Batter Ingredients:
1 c. gluten-free flour mix (130 g)
1 t. baking powder (5 g)
½ t. cinnamon (1.5 g)
1 T. refined cane sugar (optional) (13 g)
1 large egg
1 t. vanilla extract (5 ml)
2 T. pure olive oil (not extra virgin) or other neutral-flavored oil (30 ml)
1 c. hot tap water (237 ml)

Directions:
Step 1. Mix together the dry ingredients in a medium-sized mixing bowl.

Step 2. In a small bowl, whisk together the egg, vanilla extract, oil, and hot water. Add this liquid mixture to the dry ingredients. Stir well with a rubber spatula for one minute to form a smooth, thick batter that is the consistency of thick cake batter.

Step 3. Let the batter rest at room temperature for 10 minutes to activate the baking powder.

Step 4. While the batter is resting, heat the waffle iron (follow the instructions for your waffle iron during the cooking process). Use a cooking spray on the waffle iron surface before pouring half the batter (about ¾ cup or 198 g) onto the waffle iron. Cook till the waffle is golden brown and steam is no longer released from the waffle. Repeat for the second waffle.

Nutritional content: Makes 2 servings (1 waffle (243 g) per serving). Each serving contains: Calories (450); Total Fat (17 g); Saturated Fat (3 g); Cholesterol (95 mg); Sodium (680 mg); Potassium (93 mg); Total Carbohydrate (68 g); Dietary Fiber (3 g); Sugars (7 g); Protein (6 g). Nutrient(s) of note (percent of Daily Value): Vitamin A 2%, Calcium 8%, Iron 10%

Banana Pecan Chocolate Chip Waffles:

Replace the refined cane sugar in these waffles with banana for a delicious alternative. In step 1, leave out the sugar. In a separate bowl, mash one ripe banana with the back of a fork. In step 2, add the liquid ingredients to the mashed banana, and reduce the amount of hot tap water added to ¾ cup (177 ml); whisk. After thoroughly combining the liquid and dry ingredients to make the batter, add ¼ cup (45 g) mini chocolate chips (optional) and ¼ cup (25 g) chopped pecans (if tolerated). Follow steps 3 and 4 in the waffle recipe as directed.

Breakfast Cookies

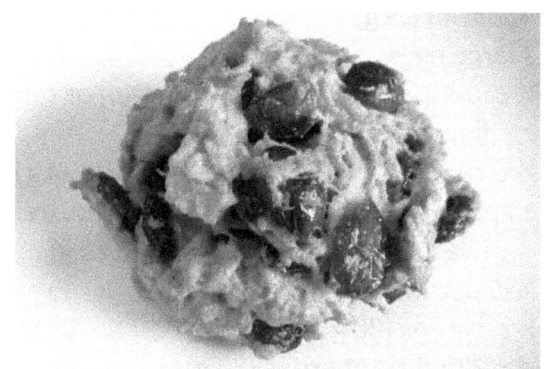

These are tasty and nutritious "cookies" that are easy to take on the go. The raisins, dried cranberries, and chopped apple keep the cookies moist. Makes about one dozen large cookies.

☑ **Allergy/Intolerance Substitutions:**
Tree nuts: In step 3, replace the pecans with shelled sunflower seeds or pumpkin seeds if tolerated.
Eggs: Prepare the equivalent of two eggs using the Flax Meal or Chia Seed Egg Replacer (pages 73 and 74), or the equivalent of one egg using the Non-rising Egg Replacer (page 76). Leave out the eggs in step 2 and add the egg replacer.
Oats: Avoid this recipe.

☑ **Reduced Sugar:**
In step 2, replace the maple syrup or honey with 50 drops of clear, alcohol-free liquid stevia, 3 T. (45 ml) milk of choice, and 1 t. (5 ml) apple cider vinegar. In step 3, leave out the dried cranberries and raisins if needed.

Dough Ingredients:
1 c. gluten-free flour mix (130 g)
1 c. certified GF rolled oats (100 g)
1 t. baking powder (5 g)
1 t. cinnamon (3 g)
¼ t. salt (1.5 g)
2 large eggs
⅓ c. pure olive oil (not extra virgin) or other neutral-flavored oil (79 ml)
⅓ c. maple syrup (79 ml) or honey (124 g)
1 apple (peeled and chopped) OR 1 c. fresh blueberries (washed and dried) (approx. 140 g)
½ c. pecans (50 g)
½ c. raisins (80 g)
½ c. dried cranberries (80 g)

Preheat Oven: 350° F/177° C

Directions:
Step 1. In a large mixing bowl, combine the gluten-free flour mix, oats, baking powder, cinnamon, and salt.

Step 2. In a small bowl, whisk together the eggs, oil, and honey or maple syrup. Add to the dry ingredients and mix with a rubber spatula till a thick dough forms.

Step 3. Add the chopped apple or blueberries, pecans, raisins, and dried cranberries. Combine thoroughly to form a thick and chunky dough.

Step 4. Line two cookie sheets with parchment paper. Spray the paper with cooking oil.

Step 5. Scoop out some dough with a large cookie dough scoop, leveling off the dough with a knife or on the edge of the mixing bowl. Release the dough ball onto a cookie sheet. Gently smooth the edge of the dough with your fingers, and flatten slightly. The cookies should be about 2 to 3 inches (5 to 8 cm) in diameter before they are placed in the oven.

Step 6. Bake for 17 to 22 minutes till golden brown. Remove the cookies from the cookie sheets with a spatula, and place on a wire rack to cool.

Nutritional content: Makes 12 servings (1 cookie (66 g) per serving; includes chopped apple). Each serving contains: Calories (180); Total Fat (5 g); Saturated Fat (0.5 g); Cholesterol (30 mg); Sodium (170 mg); Potassium (119 mg); Total Carbohydrate (33 g); Dietary Fiber (3 g); Sugars (14 g); Protein (3 g). Nutrient(s) of note (percent of Daily Value): Vitamin A 2%, Calcium 4%, Vitamin C 2%, Iron 6%

Apple Oat Muffins

Light and moist with chunks of apple, these muffins are great for breakfast -- or any time of the day! The reduced sugar version of this recipe is delicious and used frequently in my house. This recipe makes about 15 medium-sized muffins.

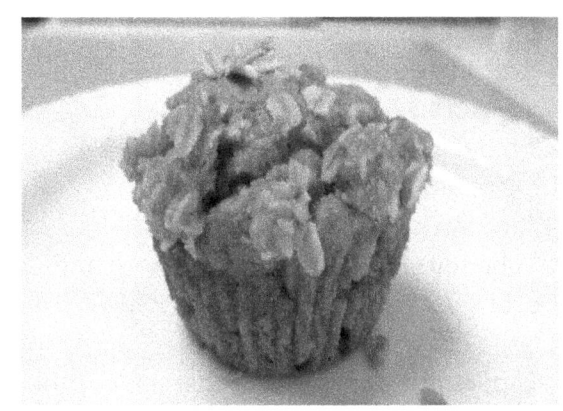

☑ **Allergy/Intolerance Substitutions:**

Eggs: Prepare the equivalent of one egg using the Rising Egg Replacer (page 74). In step 1, reduce the baking powder to 1 t. (5 g). In step 2, leave out the eggs and add the egg replacer (be sure to add the apple cider vinegar as specified in the egg replacer recipe). In step 4, fill the muffin cup liners nearly to the top.

Oats: In step 3, leave out the rolled oats; add 2 T. (13 g) flax meal, and 2 T. (13 g) of pumpkin seed meal, sunflower seed meal, *or* almond meal (as tolerated). Do not make the topping in step 5; instead, sprinkle the muffin batter with sliced almonds (if no tree nut allergy) or pumpkin seeds prior to baking.

☑ Reduced Sugar:
In step 2, leave out the sugar or honey, and add 60 drops of clear, alcohol-free liquid stevia. In step 3, leave out the raisins if needed. In step 4, fill the muffin cups almost to the top. In step 5, leave out the brown sugar and add 20 drops of liquid stevia. Makes 9 muffins.

Batter Ingredients:
1½ c. gluten-free flour mix (195 g)
1½ t. baking powder (7.5 g)
1 t. cinnamon (3 g)
½ t. nutmeg (1.5 g)
½ c. honey (174 g) or refined cane sugar (100 g)
1 c. unsweetened apple sauce (250 g)
2 large eggs
¼ c. pure olive oil (not extra virgin) or other neutral-flavored oil (59 ml)
1 t. vanilla extract (5 ml)
½ c. certified GF rolled oats (50 g)
½ c. raisins (optional) (80 g)
¼ c. chopped apple (optional) (35 g)

Topping Ingredients:
¼ c. lightly-packed brown sugar (36 g)
3 T. shortening or lard (27 g)
½ c. certified GF rolled oats (50 g)

Preheat Oven: 350° F/177° C

Directions:

Step 1. In a large mixing bowl, mix together the gluten-free flour mix, baking powder, cinnamon, and nutmeg.

Step 2. In a small bowl, whisk together the sugar or honey, apple sauce, eggs, oil, and vanilla. Add this to the dry ingredients and mix well with a rubber spatula to form a smooth, thick batter.

Step 3. Mix in the ½ cup of oats (50 g), raisins, and chopped apples till well combined.

Step 4. Place muffin liners in a muffin pan. Pour the batter carefully into each muffin liner, filling each about three-quarters full.

Step 5. For the topping, thoroughly combine the brown sugar and shortening/lard with your hands in a small mixing bowl. Mix in the ½ cup (50 g) of oats. Sprinkle about 1 Tablespoon (15 g) of this topping on the batter for each muffin.

Step 6. Place the muffin pan in the oven and bake for 22 to 25 minutes, till a toothpick inserted in the middle of the largest muffin comes out clean. Remove the pan from the oven. Let the muffins cool for 10 minutes before removing them (with muffin liners attached) from the pan.

Nutritional content: Makes 15 servings (one muffin (70 g) per serving; includes raisins and chopped apple). Each serving contains: Calories (210); Total Fat (8 g); Saturated Fat (2 g); Cholesterol (25 mg); Sodium (140 mg); Potassium (79 mg); Total Carbohydrate (34 g); Dietary Fiber (2 g); Sugars (16 g); Protein (3 g). Nutrient(s) of note (percent of Daily Value): Calcium 2%, Iron 4%

Lemon Almond Muffins

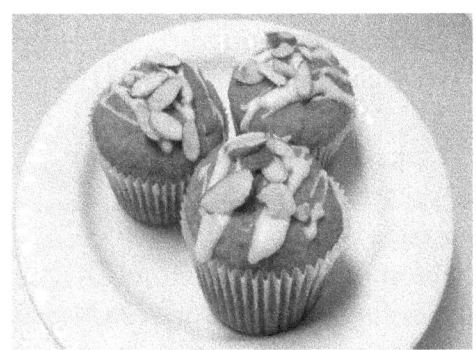

These muffins come out light and airy with a mild lemon flavor. Drizzle on a little Lemon-flavored Icing (see page 255) for an extra burst of flavor. This recipe makes 15 medium-sized muffins.

☑ **Allergy/Intolerance Substitutions:**
Tree nuts: In step 1, replace the almond meal with pumpkin seed meal or sunflower seed meal (see page 72). In step 2, replace the almond extract with vanilla extract. In step 5, replace the sliced almonds with shelled sunflower or pumpkin seeds, or leave off completely.
Eggs: Prepare the equivalent of one egg using the Rising Egg Replacer (page 74). In step 2, leave out the eggs and add the egg replacer (do *not* add the apple cider vinegar as specified in the egg replacer recipe — it is not needed because of the lemon juice).

☑ **Reduced Sugar:**
In step 2, use only 3 T. (45 ml) of lemon juice instead of the 4 T. (59 ml) listed in the original recipe; replace the honey with 60 drops of clear, alcohol-free liquid stevia, and add 1 t. (5 ml) lemon extract. In step 3, fill the muffin pan liners nearly to the top with the batter. After 15 minutes of baking, sprinkle the top of each muffin with sliced almonds

(if tolerated) and then finish baking. Do not drizzle the muffins with Lemon-flavored Icing in Step 5. Makes about 10 muffins.

Batter Ingredients:
1½ c. gluten-free flour mix (195 g)
½ c. almond meal (50 g)
1 t. baking powder (5 g)
½ c. honey (174 g)
2 large eggs
¾ c. milk of choice (177 ml)
¼ c. pure olive oil (not extra virgin) or other neutral-
    flavored oil (59 ml)
1 T. almond extract (15 ml)
Zest from two lemons
Juice from two lemons (4 T. or 59 ml)

Topping Ingredients (Optional):
Lemon-flavored Icing (see page 255)
¼ c. sliced almonds (25 g)

Preheat Oven: 350° F/177° C

Directions:
Step 1. In a large mixing bowl, mix the dry ingredients together.

Step 2. In a small mixing bowl, whisk together the honey, eggs, milk of choice, oil, almond extract, and lemon zest and juice. Add this mixture to the dry ingredients and combine well with a rubber spatula to form a smooth batter.

Step 3. Place a muffin pan liner in each cup of a muffin pan. Carefully fill each liner about two-thirds full with the batter.

Step 4. Bake for about 25 minutes, until a toothpick inserted in the center of one of the muffins comes out clean. Let the muffins cool for 15 minutes and then remove the muffins from the pan. Cool to room temperature.

Step 5. Drizzle the cooled muffins with Lemon-flavored Icing and sprinkle with sliced almonds (optional).

Nutritional content: Makes 15 servings (one muffin (57 g) per serving; excludes icing and sliced almonds). Each serving contains: Calories (150); Total Fat (7 g); Saturated Fat (1 g); Cholesterol (25 mg); Sodium (130 mg); Potassium (39 mg); Total Carbohydrate (23 g); Dietary Fiber (1 g); Sugars (9 g); Protein (2 g). Nutrient(s) of note (percent of Daily Value): Vitamin A 2%, Calcium 4%, Vitamin C 4%, Iron 4%

Fruit and Vegetable Breads

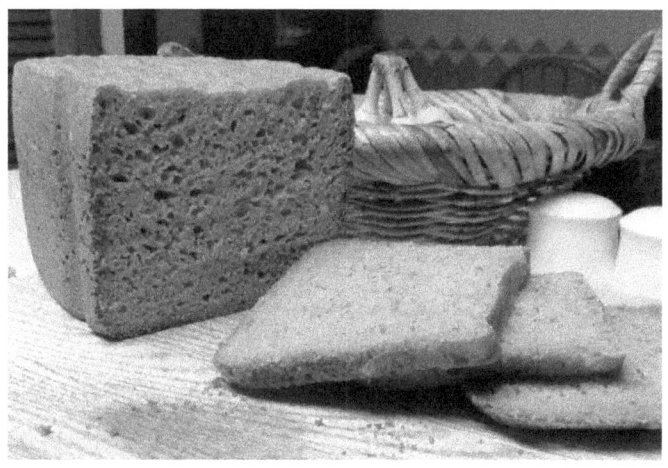

Banana Chip Bread

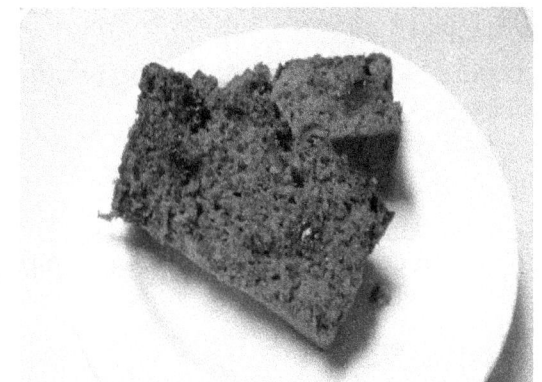

This tasty and moist bread is eaten as a dessert in my house. The flax meal adds a boost of nutrition that no one will know is there. My son really likes the addition of the chocolate chips, but leave them out for a healthier loaf.

☑ **Allergy/Intolerance Substitutions:**
Tree nuts: Leave out the pecans in step 4.
Eggs: Prepare the equivalent of two eggs using the Rising Egg Replacer (page 74). Leave out the eggs in step 2, and add the egg replacer (be sure to add the apple cider vinegar as directed in the egg replacer recipe).

☑ **Reduced Sugar:**
In step 2, leave out the honey; add 50 drops of clear, alcohol-free liquid stevia, and 2 t. (10 ml) of apple cider vinegar (do not add this vinegar if using the Rising Egg Replacer, as the egg replacer already includes apple cider vinegar). In step 4, leave out the chocolate chips, or use sugar-free GF-DF-SF chocolate or carob chips.

Batter Ingredients:
1¼ c. gluten-free flour mix (162 g)
1 t. baking powder (5 g)
¼ c. flax meal (26 g)
2 very ripe medium-sized bananas
2 large eggs
¼ c. milk of choice (59 ml)
¼ c. pure olive oil (not extra virgin) or other neutral-flavored oil (59 ml)
½ c. honey (174 g)
1 t. vanilla extract (5 ml)
½ c. chopped pecans (optional) (50 g)
½ c. GF-DF-SF chocolate chips (optional) (90 g)

Preheat Oven: 350° F/177° C

Directions:
Step 1. In a medium-sized bowl, mix together the gluten-free flour mix, baking powder, and flax.

Step 2. In a large mixing bowl, thoroughly mash the bananas with the back of a fork or a potato masher. Add the eggs, milk of choice, oil, honey, and vanilla extract; mix well.

Step 3. Add the dry ingredients to the banana mixture. Using a rubber spatula, mix all of the ingredients together to form a smooth, thick batter (it is okay if there are some small chunks of banana in the batter).

Step 4. Fold in the chopped pecans and chocolate chips.

Step 5. Spray an 8" x 4" (20 cm x 10 cm) medium-sized loaf pan with cooking oil. Pour the batter into the pan, spreading the batter into the corners with the rubber spatula. Bake for 55 to 65 minutes till a toothpick inserted in the center of the bread comes out clean.

Step 6. Cool for 15 minutes. Remove the bread from the pan and place it on a cooling rack. Cool for 45 minutes more before slicing. This bread can also be eaten warm right from the pan.

Nutritional content: Makes 12 servings (1 slice (74 g) per serving; includes pecans and excludes chocolate chips). Each serving contains: Calories (210); Total Fat (10 g); Saturated Fat (1 g); Cholesterol (30 mg); Sodium (135 mg); Potassium (123 mg); Total Carbohydrate (30 g); Dietary Fiber (2 g); Sugars (14 g); Protein (3 g). Nutrient(s) of note (percent of Daily Value): Vitamin A 2%, Calcium 2%, Vitamin C 4%, Iron 4%

Pumpkin Bread

If you don't like pumpkin bread, this recipe will change your mind. This cake-like bread comes out very moist and delicious, and disappears from my kitchen counter usually within a few hours. I make this family favorite in the fall when I can get pumpkins fresh from a local farm. You can replace the pumpkin in this recipe with unsweetened apple sauce to make an equally good apple bread! To serve this bread as a dessert, top it with a little Cashew-Coconut Cream Topping or some Frozen Coconut Vanilla Custard (see the last chapter for these recipes).

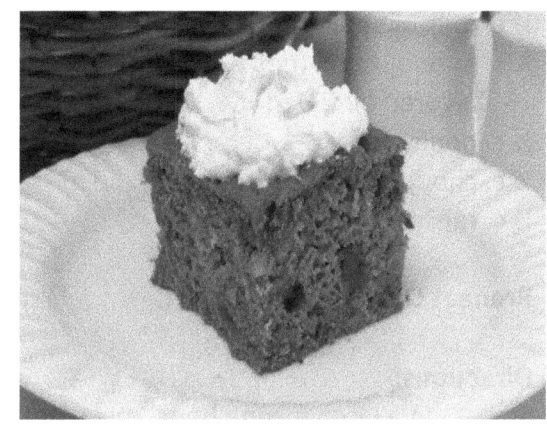

☑ **Allergy/Intolerance Substitutions:**
Tree nuts: Leave out the pecans in Step 3.
Eggs: No suggestions given; this recipe does not work well with egg replacer.

☑ **Reduced Sugar:**
No suggestions given; this recipe does not work well without honey.

Batter Ingredients:
1¼ c. gluten-free flour mix (162 g)
1 t. baking powder (5 g)
1 t. cinnamon (3 g)
1 c. canned or fresh pumpkin (roasted and pureed; 240 g)
2 large eggs
½ c. milk of choice (118 ml)
¼ c. pure olive oil (not extra virgin) or other neutral-flavored oil (59 ml)
½ c. honey (174 g)
½ c. chopped pecans (optional) (50 g)
½ c. raisins (optional) (80 g)

Preheat Oven: 350° F/177° C

Directions:
Step 1. In a large mixing bowl, mix together the gluten-free flour mix, baking powder, and cinnamon.

Step 2. In a small mixing bowl, whisk together the pumpkin, eggs, milk of choice, oil, and honey. Add to the dry ingredients, and mix well with a rubber spatula to form a smooth, thick batter.

Step 3. Fold the pecans and raisins into the batter.

Step 4. Spray an 8" x 8" (20 cm x 20 cm) square pan with cooking oil. Pour the batter into the pan, spreading the batter into the corners with a rubber spatula. Bake for about 35 to 40 minutes or until a toothpick inserted in the center of the bread comes out clean. Cool to room temperature or serve warm directly from the pan.

Nutritional content: Makes 9 servings (one square piece (84 g) per serving; includes pecans and raisins). Each serving contains: Calories (200); Total Fat (9 g); Saturated Fat (1 g); Cholesterol (30 mg); Sodium (140 mg); Potassium (148 mg); Total Carbohydrate (31 g); Dietary Fiber (2 g); Sugars (15 g); Protein (3 g). Nutrient(s) of note (percent of Daily Value): Vitamin A 25%, Calcium 4%, Vitamin C 2%, Iron 4%

Roasting a Pumpkin:

Slice the pumpkin in half, scrape out the seeds with a large metal spoon, place the pumpkin halves cut-side down in a baking pan, and bake at 375° F (191° C) for about one hour till soft. Remove from the oven and cool. Scrape the pumpkin out of its shell, and puree with a wand blender or other blender; use as directed in the recipe. Freeze any extra pureed pumpkin in 1 cup (240 g) portions in freezer bags or freezer-safe glass jars for future recipes.

Zucchini Bread

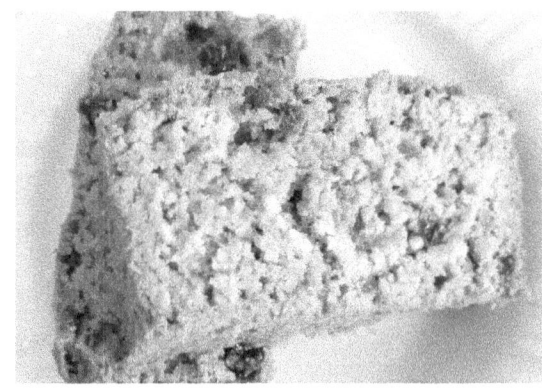

This recipe is for those who want something tasty and nutritious at the same time. The almond meal boosts the protein in this loaf, while the flax adds omega-3 and fiber. Frozen and thawed zucchini works well with the original recipe, but does not work well for the egg substitution and reduced sugar recipes (use fresh zucchini only when making these substitutions).

☑ Allergy/Intolerance Substitutions:

Tree nuts: In step 1, replace the almond meal with quinoa flour, pumpkin seed meal, or sunflower seed meal. In step 3, leave out the pecans.

Eggs: Use fresh zucchini only when using egg replacer. Prepare the egg replacement equivalent of two eggs using the Rising Egg Replacer (page 74). In step 2, leave out the eggs and add the egg replacer (be sure to add the apple cider vinegar as specified in the egg replacer recipe).

☑ **Reduced Sugar:**
Use fresh zucchini only. In step 1, add an additional ½ t. (1.5 g) cinnamon (i.e., 1½ t. or 4.5 g cinnamon total). In step 2, replace the honey with 50 drops of clear, alcohol-free liquid stevia and ⅓ cup (83 g) unsweetened applesauce. In step 3, leave out the raisins if needed.

Batter Ingredients:
1½ c. gluten-free flour mix (195 g)
1 t. baking powder (5 g)
¼ c. almond meal (25 g)
¼ c. flax meal (26 g)
1 t. cinnamon (3 g)
¼ t. ground nutmeg (0.8 g)
1 cup shredded zucchini, lightly packed (140 g)
2 large eggs
½ c. milk of choice (118 ml)
⅓ c. pure olive oil (not extra virgin) or other neutral-flavored oil (79 ml)
½ c. honey (174 g)
½ c. chopped pecans (optional) (50 g)
½ c. raisins (80 g)

Preheat Oven: 350° F/177° C

Directions:

Step 1. In a large mixing bowl, mix the dry ingredients together.

Step 2. In a medium-sized bowl, whisk together the shredded zucchini, eggs, milk of choice, oil, and honey. Add this mixture to the dry ingredients; mix with a rubber spatula to form a thick batter.

Step 3. Fold the pecans and raisins into the batter.

Step 4. Spray an 8" x 4" (20 cm x 10 cm) medium-sized loaf pan with cooking spray. Pour the batter into the pan. Bake for 55 to 65 minutes or until a toothpick inserted in the center of the loaf comes out clean. Cool for 15 minutes. Remove from the pan and place on a cooling rack. Cool for 45 minutes more before slicing. This bread can also be eaten warm right from the pan.

Nutritional content: Makes 12 servings (one slice (83 g) per serving; includes pecans and raisins). Each serving contains: Calories (250); Total Fat (13 g); Saturated Fat (1.5 g); Cholesterol (30 mg); Sodium (160 mg); Potassium (131 mg); Total Carbohydrate (34 g); Dietary Fiber (3 g); Sugars (15 g); Protein (4 g). Nutrient(s) of note (percent of Daily Value): Vitamin A 2%, Calcium 4%, Vitamin C 4%, Iron 6%

Carrot Spice Bread

This moist, nutritious, and delicious bread has a little spice courtesy of the ground ginger and cayenne. It goes well with any dinner, and is equally good as a snack.

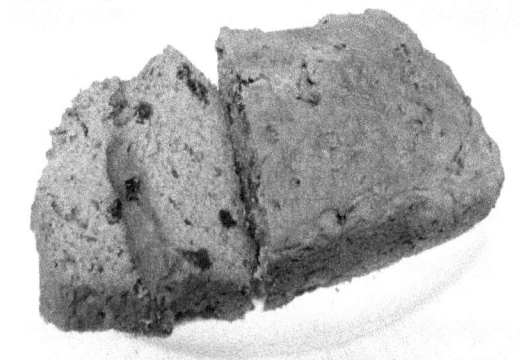

☑ **Allergy/Intolerance Substitutions:**
Tree nuts: In step 1, replace the almond meal with quinoa flour, pumpkin seed meal, or sunflower seed meal. In step 3, leave out the pecans.
Eggs: Prepare the equivalent of two eggs using the Rising Egg Replacer (page 74). In step 2, leave out the eggs and add the egg replacer (add the apple cider vinegar as specified in the egg replacer recipe).
Nightshade family: In step 1, leave out the cayenne pepper.

☑ **Reduced Sugar:**
In step 1, add an additional ½ t. (1.5 g) cinnamon (i.e., 1½ t. or 4.5 g cinnamon total). In step 2, replace the honey with 50 drops of clear, alcohol-free liquid stevia and ¼ cup (62 g) unsweetened applesauce. In step 3, leave out the raisins if needed.

Batter Ingredients:
1½ c. gluten-free flour mix (195 g)
1 t. baking powder (5 g)
¼ c. almond meal or quinoa flour (25 g)
¼ c. flax meal (26 g)
1 t. cinnamon (3 g)
1½ t. ground dried ginger (4.5 g)
½ t. ground nutmeg (1.5 g)
¼ t. ground dried cayenne pepper (0.7 g)
¼ t. salt (1.5 g)
1½ c. shredded carrot, lightly packed (210 g)
2 large eggs
1 c. milk of choice (237 ml)
⅓ c. pure olive oil (not extra virgin) or other neutral-flavored oil (79 ml)
⅓ c. honey (124 g)
½ c. chopped pecans (optional) (50 g)
½ c. raisins (80 g)

Preheat Oven: 350° F/177° C

Directions:
Step 1. In a large mixing bowl, mix the dry ingredients (including the spices) together.

Step 2. In a medium-sized mixing bowl, whisk together the shredded carrot, eggs, milk of choice, oil, and honey. Add this mixture to the dry ingredients; mix with a rubber spatula to form a thick batter.

Step 3. Fold the pecans and raisins into the batter.
Step 4. Spray an 8" x 4" (20 cm x 10 cm) medium-sized loaf pan with cooking spray. Pour the batter into the pan and smooth the top of it with a rubber spatula. Bake for 55

to 65 minutes or until a toothpick Inserted in the center of the loaf comes out clean. Cool for 15 minutes. Remove from the pan and place on a cooling rack. Cool for 45 minutes more before slicing. This bread can also be eaten warm right from the pan.

Nutritional content: Makes 12 servings (one slice (91 g) per serving; includes pecans and raisins). Each serving contains: Calories (240); Total Fat (13 g); Saturated Fat (1.5 g); Cholesterol (30 mg); Sodium (220 mg); Potassium (157 mg); Total Carbohydrate (31 g); Dietary Fiber (3 g); Sugars (12 g); Protein (4 g). Nutrient(s) of note (percent of Daily Value): Vitamin A 50%, Calcium 6%, Vitamin C 2%, Iron 6%

Corn Bread with a Kick

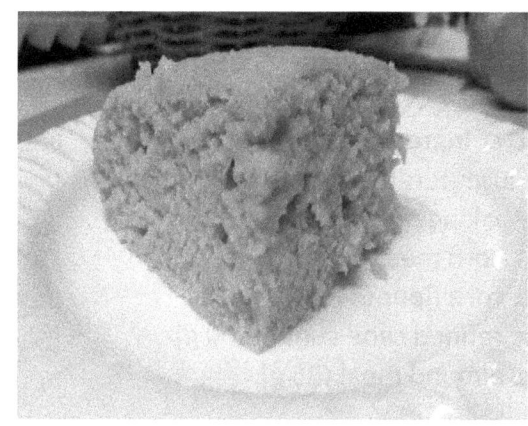

C reating a GF-DF-SF corn bread that is moist is a challenge since butter normally keeps corn bread moist. Adding a small amount of almond meal keeps the moisture high and also adds a little sweetness. If you like a little spice in corn bread, add the hot pepper sauce and green chilies; adding a few tablespoons of hot pepper jelly in place of the hot pepper sauce is excellent as well. For an unsweetened cornbread suitable for poultry stuffing, follow the "reduced sugar" directions but leave out the stevia.

☑ **Allergy/Intolerance Substitutions:**

Corn: Avoid this recipe.

Tree nuts: In step 1, replace the almond meal with pumpkin seed meal or sunflower seed meal (see page 72).

Eggs: Prepare the equivalent of one egg using the Rising Egg Replacer (page 74). In step 2, leave out the egg and add the egg replacer (be sure to add the apple cider vinegar as specified in the egg replacer recipe).

Nightshade family: In step 2, leave out the hot pepper sauce. In step 3, leave out the green chilies or jalapeño.

☑ **Reduced Sugar:**
In step 1, leave out the sugar. In step 2, reduce the amount of milk of choice added to ½ cup (118 ml); add ½ cup (125 g) unsweetened applesauce, 1 t. (5 ml) apple cider vinegar, and 70 drops of clear, alcohol-free liquid stevia. (Note: if using Rising Egg Replacer in combination with this reduced sugar recipe, you will add a total of 2 t. (10 ml) of apple cider vinegar).

Batter Ingredients:
1½ c. gluten-free flour mix (195 g)
1 t. baking powder (5 g)
½ c. corn meal (66 g)
¼ c. corn flour (31 g)
½ c. refined cane sugar (100 g)
¼ c. almond meal (25 g)
½ t. salt (3 g)
1 large egg
1 c. milk of choice (237 ml)
½ c. pure olive oil (not extra virgin) or other neutral-flavored oil (118 ml)
½ t. hot pepper sauce (optional) (2.5 ml)
½ c. fresh, raw corn kernels (optional) (70 g)
1 can (4.5 ounces or 127 g) chopped green chilies, well drained, OR one fresh minced jalapeño (optional)

Preheat Oven: 350° F/177° C

Directions:

Step 1. Mix the dry ingredients together in a large mixing bowl.

Step 2. In a small mixing bowl, whisk together the egg, milk of choice, olive oil, and hot pepper sauce. Add to the dry ingredients, and mix well with a rubber spatula to form a somewhat smooth, gritty batter.

Step 3. Fold in the corn kernels, and green chilies or chopped jalapeño (optional).

Step 4. Spray a square 8" x 8" (20 cm x 20 cm) baking pan with cooking oil. Spread the batter evenly in the pan. Bake for 25 to 30 minutes, until the top is golden brown and a toothpick inserted in the center comes out clean. Serve warm from the pan.

Nutritional content: Makes 9 servings (one square piece (101 g) per serving; includes corn kernels; excludes hot pepper sauce and chilies/jalapeño). Each serving contains: Calories (310); Total Fat (16 g); Saturated Fat (2 g); Cholesterol (20 mg); Sodium (340 mg); Potassium (97 mg); Total Carbohydrate (42 g); Dietary Fiber (2 g); Sugars (13 g); Protein (4 g). Nutrient(s) of note (percent of Daily Value): Vitamin A 2%, Calcium 4%, Iron 6%

Applesauce Sandwich Bread

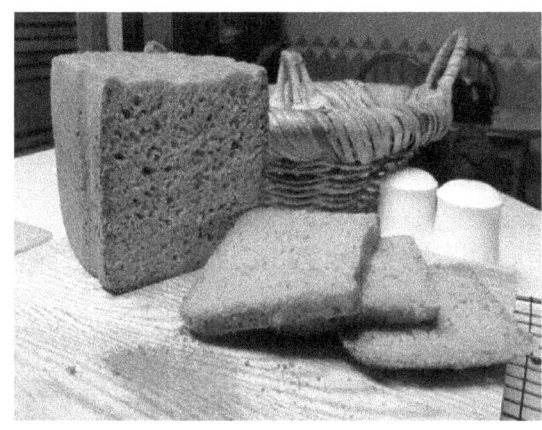

This bread is great hot out of the oven, sliced and toasted, or in stuffing recipes. The applesauce in this bread does not overpower the taste, but keeps the bread moist and flavorful. The oat flour keeps the bread firm. You can easily make your own oat flour by food-processing certified GF rolled oats until a powder forms. I like the taste of the maple syrup in this recipe, but you can use honey as a replacement for the syrup if maple products are not readily available in your area. I use a bread machine to bake this bread, but you can adapt the recipe for baking in an oven as well.

☑ Allergy/Intolerance Substitutions:

Eggs: Prepare the egg replacer equivalent of three eggs, two made using the Rising Egg Replacer (page 74) and one from the Flax Meal Egg Replacer (page 73). In step 3, leave out the eggs and add the three egg replacers. Be sure to add the apple cider vinegar as directed in the Rising Egg Replacer recipe; you will add 3 t. (15 ml) of apple cider vinegar total to this recipe since one teaspoon (5 ml) is already included in the original recipe. If intolerant of flax, add 2 T. (30 ml) milk of choice instead of the Flax Meal Egg Replacer.

Oats: In step 1, replace the oat flour with the following: 2 T. (13 g) flax meal (i.e., in addition to the 2 T. (13 g) flax meal already included in the recipe); 2 T. (13 g) almond meal, pumpkin seed meal, or sunflower seed meal; and 1/4 cup (30 g) amaranth flour.

Yeast: Avoid this recipe.

☑ Reduced Sugar:
No suggestions given; this bread will not rise well without the addition of the molasses, maple syrup, or honey.

Dough Ingredients:
2¼ t. rapid rise yeast (1 packet; 9 g)
2 c. gluten-free flour mix (260 g)
½ c. certified GF oat flour (58 g)
½ c. arrowroot starch or tapioca starch (60 g)
2 T. flax meal (13 g)
1½ t. salt (9 g)
3 large eggs
⅓ c. smooth, unsweetened applesauce (83 g)
¼ c. pure olive oil (not extra virgin) or other neutral-flavored oil (59 ml)
¼ c. maple syrup (59 ml) or honey (87 g)
1 T. molasses (15 ml)
1 t. apple cider vinegar (5 ml)
⅔ c. hot tap or filtered water (105-115° F or 40-46°C; 158 ml)

Directions:

Step 1. Place the yeast in the yeast compartment of your bread machine.

Step 2. In a large mixing bowl, mix together the gluten-free flour mix, oat flour, arrowroot or tapioca starch, flax meal, and salt.

Step 3. In a separate mixing bowl, whisk together the remaining ingredients till well combined. Add this liquid mixture to the flour mixture and combine thoroughly with a rubber spatula. Pour into the pan of the bread machine. (NOTE: I usually mix the wet and dry ingredients together *before* putting them into the bread machine since bread machines do not always adequately mix the ingredients due to the heaviness of the gluten-free flours.)

Step 4. Set your bread machine for baking a large loaf and for the desired crust texture. Start the bread machine.

Step 5. When the baking cycle is finished, promptly remove the loaf from the pan and place on a cooling rack. Cool for two hours before slicing.

Nutritional content: Make 12 servings (1 slice (85 g) per serving). Each serving contains: Calories (220); Total Fat (7 g); Saturated Fat (1 g); Cholesterol (45 mg); Sodium (430 mg); Potassium (96 mg); Total Carbohydrate (35 g); Dietary Fiber (2 g); Sugars (6 g); Protein (4 g). Nutrient(s) of note (percent of Daily Value): Vitamin A 2%, Calcium 2%, Iron 6%

Home-style Poultry Stuffing

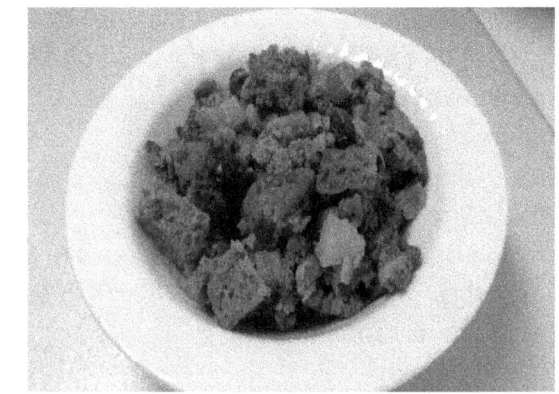

Prior to using homemade bread in my poultry stuffing, my gluten-free stuffing was truly horrible (just ask my family). The secret to good gluten-free stuffing is using a good, fresh (not stale) loaf of GF bread and whatever secret ingredients your family traditionally adds. Depending on the amount of additional ingredients added, this stuffing will generally serve about twelve light eaters; double the recipe for additional guests. Crumble the leftover bread crusts into bread crumbs and freeze in a zipper bag for other recipes.

☑ **Allergy/Intolerance Substitutions:**
Eggs: Prepare the equivalent of one egg using the Non-rising, Flax Meal, or Chia Seed Egg Replacer recipe (pages 73-76). In step 6, leave out the egg and add the egg replacer.
Yeast: Use a yeast-free bread.

☑ **Reduced Sugar:**
In step 1, use an unsweetened bread. In step 5, use an unsweetened sausage. In step 6, leave out the dried cranberries if needed.

Preparation the Day Before:
Make one loaf of Applesauce-Oat Sandwich Bread or other bread of choice.

Stuffing Ingredients:
One loaf of Applesauce-Oat Sandwich Bread or other bread of choice
2 T. olive oil or other neutral-flavored oil (30 ml)
1 medium onion, chopped
3 celery stalks, chopped
1 green apple, peeled and chopped
3 T. of chopped fresh sage (6 g)
1 pound of GF-DF-SF loose Italian sausage (453 g)
1 large egg
½ c. of dried cranberries (80 g)
Salt and pepper
1 to 2 cups GF-DF-SF chicken broth or vegetable broth (237 to 473 ml)

Preheat Oven: 325° F/163° C

Directions:
Step 1. Use a serrated bread knife to remove the crust from the cooled loaf of bread. Cut the loaf into ¾-inch (2 cm) cubes, and place them on an 11" x 13" (28 cm x 33 cm) baking pan.

Step 2. Bake the cubes for 60 to 80 minutes, turning them every 15 minutes with a metal spatula, till all sides of the cubes are dry and crisp to the touch. Do not air-dry the cubes as stale gluten-free bread will not re-soften the same as stale wheat bread when the stuffing ingredients are mixed together.

Step 3. Pour the bread cubes into a large mixing bowl and let them cool to room temperature. Follow your traditional stuffing recipe or continue with the recipe below.

Step 4. Pour 2 Tablespoons (30 ml) of olive oil into a large frying pan. Over medium heat, sauté together the chopped onion, chopped celery, and chopped green apple, until the onions become translucent and the celery has softened slightly (about 5 to 10 minutes). Add the chopped sage and sauté for one minute more. Pour this mixture into the large mixing bowl with the bread cubes.

Step 5. Place the loose sausage in the frying pan. Cook the sausage over medium heat, flipping it with a spatula, until it is completely cooked through. As it cooks, cut it into bite-sized pieces using a fork and knife. Transfer the cooked sausage to a bowl that has been lined with paper towel, and let the sausage drain for a few minutes.

Step 6. To the large mixing bowl, add the cooked Italian sausage, raw egg, dried cranberries, and a little salt and pepper (if the broth or the sausage is already salted, you may need to reduce the amount of salt added). Use a large metal or wooden spoon to gently combine all the ingredients (try not to break the bread cubes as you mix).

Step 7. Slowly add ½ cup (118 ml) of the broth, pouring it in a thin stream over the entire mixture. Using the metal or wooden spoon, gently combine the broth with the stuffing mixture. Let the mixture sit for one minute to absorb the liquid. Repeat this process, adding another ½ cup (118 ml) of the broth. Check the bread cubes to see if enough broth has been added (the outside of the cubes should be slightly mushy while the inside remains somewhat firm.) If more broth is needed, add ¼ cup (59 ml) at a time, gently mixing the ingredients together after each addition, until the cubes have been adequately moistened. Be careful not to add too much broth as the bread cubes will become soggy.

Step 8. For a moist stuffing, bake the stuffing in a slow cooker on low for about 3 hours, until the stuffing reaches an internal temperature of 165° F (74° C). For a stuffing with a crisp top, bake as follows: Pre-heat the oven to 350° F (177° C). Spray a large (84 oz. or 2.5 liter) casserole dish with cooking oil. Pour the stuffing into the casserole dish and cover. Bake for 40 minutes. Remove the cover of the casserole dish and bake approximately ten minutes more, until the stuffing reaches an internal temperature of 165° F (74° C).

Nutritional content: Makes 12 servings (¾ cup per serving or 208 g; includes all ingredients listed in recipe, including Applesauce-Oat Bread). Each serving contains: Calories (340); Total Fat (13 g); Saturated Fat (3 g); Cholesterol (60 mg); Sodium (700 mg); Potassium (282 mg); Total Carbohydrate (45 g); Dietary Fiber (3 g); Sugars (13 g); Protein (11 g). Nutrient(s) of note (percent of Daily Value): Vitamin A 4%, Calcium 4%, Vitamin C 4%, Iron 8%

Cakes and Other Desserts

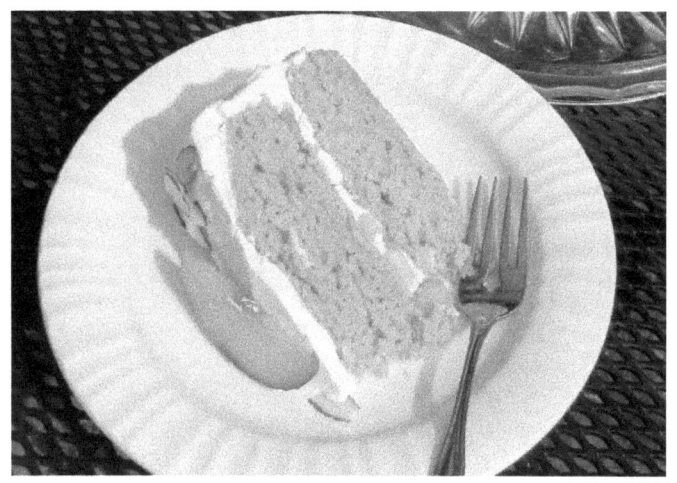

Simple Yellow Cake

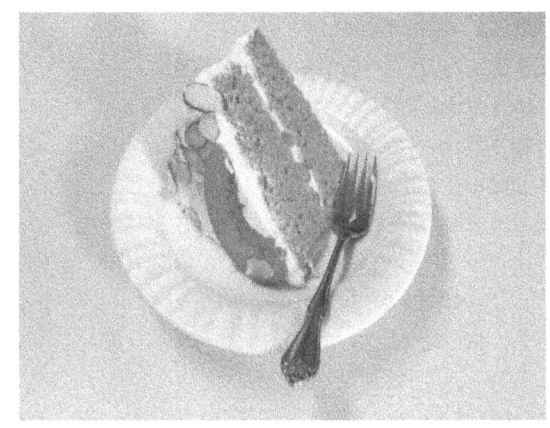

Moist and rich, this cake can be used with any type of frosting you choose (recipes for frostings can be found in the last chapter) or with fresh fruit. This recipe makes one 8" or 9" (20 cm or 23 cm) diameter cake layer; double the recipe for two layers (shown in photo) or a 13" x 9" (33 cm x 23 cm) sheet pan. You can also use this recipe to make cupcakes (fill muffin cups ⅔ full and shorten the baking time slightly).

☑ Allergy/Intolerance Substitutions:
Eggs: Prepare the egg replacer equivalent of two eggs using the Rising Egg Replacer (page 74). In step 2, leave out the eggs and add the egg replacer (be sure to add the apple cider vinegar as directed in the egg replacer recipe).

☑ Reduced Sugar:
In step 1, leave out the sugar and add 1 T. (4.5 g) coconut flour (if tolerated). In step 2, add 75 drops of clear, alcohol-free liquid stevia and 1 t. (5 ml) apple cider vinegar (do not add this teaspoon of vinegar if using the Rising Egg Replacer, as apple cider vinegar is already included in the

egg replacer recipe). In step 3, pour the batter into the cake pan and spread evenly with a rubber spatula. Brush the top of the batter with a pastry brush dipped in a little egg white or olive oil to completely smooth. Bake as directed.

Batter Ingredients:
1½ c. gluten-free flour mix (195 g)
½ c. refined cane sugar (100 g)
1 t. baking powder (5 g)
2 large eggs
½ c. milk of choice (118 ml)
⅓ c. pure olive oil (not extra virgin) or other neutral-flavored oil (79 ml)
1 T. vanilla extract (15 ml)

Preheat Oven: 350° F/177° C

Directions:
Step 1. In a large mixing bowl, combine the dry ingredients.

Step 2. In a small mixing bowl, whisk together the eggs, milk, oil, and vanilla extract. Add to the dry ingredients and mix well with a rubber spatula to form a smooth, thick batter.

Step 3. Spray an 8" or 9" (20 cm or 23 cm) round cake pan or 8" x 8" (20 cm x 20 cm) square pan with cooking oil. Pour the batter into the pan and spread it evenly with a rubber spatula, smoothing the top.

Step 4. Bake for about 20 to 25 minutes, until a toothpick inserted in the center comes out clean; do not over bake.

Step 5. Let the cake cool for 20 minutes and then remove it from the pan. Cool the cake completely before frosting.

Nutritional content: Makes 12 servings (1 slice (52 g) per serving; toppings excluded). Each serving contains: Calories (170); Total Fat (7 g); Saturated Fat (1 g); Cholesterol (30 mg); Sodium (150 mg); Potassium (34 mg); Total Carbohydrate (24 g); Dietary Fiber (1 g); Sugars (9 g); Protein (2 g). Nutrient(s) of note (percent of Daily Value): Vitamin A 2%, Calcium 2%, Iron 2%

Rich Chocolate Cake

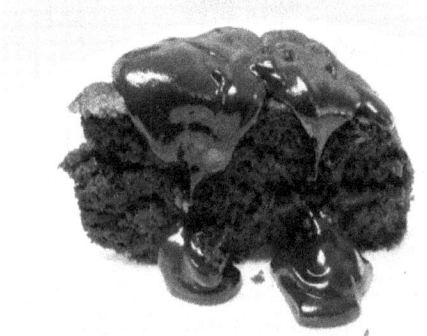

This cake is simple to make but rich in flavor. This recipe makes one 8" or 9" (20 cm or 23 cm) diameter round cake layer; double the recipe for two layers or a 9" x 13" (23 cm x 33 cm) sheet pan. You can also use this recipe to make cupcakes (you may need to shorten the baking time). Use the Cashew Coconut Cream topping (page 245) between layers and Chocolate Coconut Frosting (page 249) on top, or cover with warm Chocolate Coconut Ganache (page 249; see photo).

☑ **Allergy/Intolerance Substitutions:**
Eggs: Prepare the equivalent of two eggs using the Rising Egg Replacer (page 74). In step 2, leave out the eggs and add the egg replacer (be sure to add the apple cider vinegar as specified in the egg replacer recipe).

☑ **Reduced Sugar:**
In step 1, leave out the sugar; add ¼ cup (25 g) of almond meal, pumpkin seed meal, or sunflower seed meal (as tolerated) to the dry ingredients. In step 2, leave out the milk of choice; add 65 drops of clear, alcohol-free liquid stevia, ½ cup (125 g) unsweetened apple sauce, and 1 t. (5

ml) apple cider vinegar (do not add this apple cider vinegar if using the Rising Egg Replacer since apple cider vinegar is already included in the egg replacer recipe). In step 3, after smoothing the top of the batter with a rubber spatula, smooth further using a pastry brush dipped in either egg white or olive oil.

Batter Ingredients:
1¼ c. gluten-free flour mix (162 g)
½ c. GF-DF-SF unsweetened cocoa powder (50 g)
½ c. refined cane sugar (100 g)
1 t. baking powder (5 g)
2 large eggs
1 c. milk of choice (237 ml)
½ c. pure olive oil (not extra virgin) or other neutral-flavored oil (118 ml)
1 t. vanilla extract (5 ml)

Preheat Oven: 350° F/177° C

Directions:
Step 1. In a large mixing bowl, mix the dry ingredients with a rubber spatula till the cocoa and flour are completely combined.

Step 2. In a small bowl, whisk together the eggs, milk of choice, oil, and vanilla extract. Add this mixture to the dry ingredients and stir well with a rubber spatula to form a smooth, thick batter.

Step 3. Spray an 8" or 9" (20 cm or 23 cm) round cake pan or 8" x 8" (20 cm x 20 cm) square pan with cooking oil. Pour the batter into the pan and spread it evenly with a rubber spatula, smoothing the top.

Step 4. Bake for 20 to 25 minutes, until a toothpick inserted in the center comes out clean; do not over bake.

Step 5. Let the cake cool for 20 minutes and then remove it from the pan. Cool the cake completely before frosting.

Nutritional content: Makes 12 servings (1 slice (65 g) per serving; toppings excluded). Each serving contains: Calories (190); Total Fat (11 g); Saturated Fat (2 g); Cholesterol (30 mg); Sodium (150 mg); Potassium (93 mg); Total Carbohydrate (24 g); Dietary Fiber (2 g); Sugars (9 g); Protein (2 g). Nutrient(s) of note (percent of Daily Value): Vitamin A 2%, Calcium 4%, Iron 6%

Moist Almond Crumb Cake

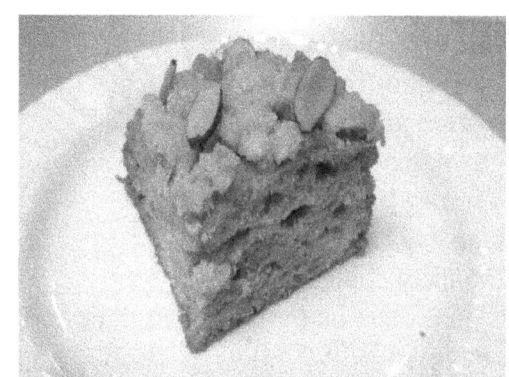

This cake is great with a cup of coffee or tea. The crumb topping adds a little crunch to the moist cake. For a sweeter treat, drizzle on Vanilla-flavored Icing (see page 255), or serve with some Frozen Coconut Vanilla Custard (page 257).

☑ **Allergy/Intolerance Substitutions:**
Tree nuts: Avoid this recipe.
Eggs: In one bowl, prepare the equivalent of two eggs using the Rising Egg Replacer (page 74). In a second bowl, prepare the equivalent of one egg using the Non-rising Egg Replacer (page 76). In step 2, for the batter, leave out the eggs and add 5 T. (75 ml) of the Rising Egg Replacer (add 2 t. or 10 ml apple cider vinegar directly to the batter instead of to the egg replacer as specified in the Rising Egg Replacer recipe). In step 3, for the crumb topping, replace the egg white with 3 T. (45 ml) of the Non-rising Egg Replacer.

☑ **Reduced Sugar:**
In step 2, replace the honey with 40 drops of clear, alcohol-free liquid stevia, ⅓ cup (83 g) unsweetened applesauce, and 1 t. (5 ml) apple cider vinegar (leave the

vinegar out if using Rising Egg Replacer since the replacer already includes vinegar). For the crumb topping (step 3), replace the sugar with 50 drops of liquid stevia and add an extra ½ t. (1.5 g) cinnamon (i.e., 1 t. or 3 g of cinnamon total).

Batter Ingredients:
1½ c. gluten-free flour mix (195 g)
½ c. almond meal (50 g)
1 t. baking powder (5 g)
¼ c. honey (87 g)
2 large eggs
½ c. milk of choice (118 ml)
⅓ c. pure olive oil (not extra virgin) or other neutral-flavored oil (79 ml)
1 T. almond extract (15 ml)

Crumb Topping Ingredients:
¾ c. almond meal (75 g)
½ c. refined cane sugar (100 g)
½ c. gluten-free flour mix (65 g)
½ t. cinnamon (1.5 g)
1 egg white
2 to 3 T. shortening or lard (18 to 27 g)
¼ c. sliced almonds (25 g)

Preheat Oven: 350° F/177° C

Directions:

Step 1. For the batter, mix together the 1½ cups (195 g) gluten-free flour mix, ½ cup almond meal (50 g), and baking powder in a large mixing bowl.

Step 2. In a small mixing bowl, whisk together the honey, two eggs, milk of choice, oil, and almond extract. Add this mixture to the dry ingredients, mixing well with a rubber spatula to form a smooth batter.

Step 3. For the crumb topping, mix together the ¾ cup (75 g) almond meal, sugar, ½ cup (65 g) gluten-free flour mix, and cinnamon in a small mixing bowl. Add the egg white and 2 T. (18 g) of shortening or lard; combine the ingredients with your hands till no lumps of shortening/lard can be seen. The crumb topping should be slightly sticky in texture. Test the crumbs by squeezing some in your hands; if large crumbs form and don't fall apart, the crumbs contain the correct amount of shortening/lard. If crumbs do not form, add one additional tablespoon (9 g) of shortening/lard, and mix into the crumb mixture; re-test the crumbs to see if they hold together when squeezed.

Step 4. Spray an 8" x 8" (20 cm x 20 cm) square pan or 8" (20 cm) round cake pan with cooking oil. Pour the batter into the pan and spread it evenly with a rubber spatula.

Step 5. Squeeze the topping mixture into pea-sized (or larger) crumbs with your hands as you sprinkle the crumbs on top of the batter.

Step 6. Bake for 20 minutes. With the cake still in the oven, sprinkle the sliced almonds on top of the crumbs.

Step 7. Bake for 15 to 20 minutes more, until a toothpick inserted in the center comes out clean and the crumbs are lightly browned. Let the cake cool to room temperature. Serve straight from the pan.

Nutritional content: Makes 9 servings (1 square piece (115 g) per serving). Each serving contains: Calories (410); Total Fat (22 g); Saturated Fat (3.5 g); Cholesterol (40 mg); Sodium (260 mg); Potassium (83 mg); Total Carbohydrate (50 g); Dietary Fiber (3 g); Sugars (20 g); Protein (7 g). Nutrient(s) of note (percent of Daily Value): Vitamin A 2%, Calcium 8%, Iron 8%

Blueberry Crumb Cake

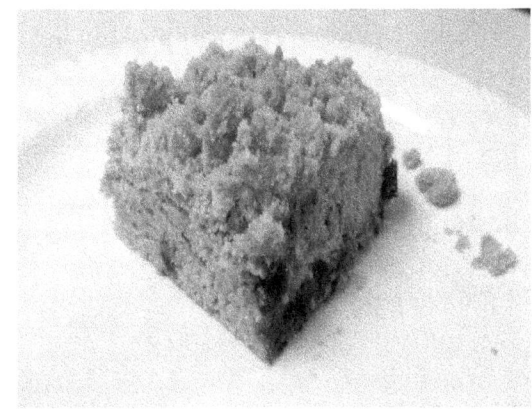

This recipe is a favorite of my friends. It is so tasty that you will make it frequently. This recipe works best with fresh blueberries (the batter does not rise correctly when frozen blueberries are used, and folding thawed blueberries into the batter turns it blue). Serve warm with Frozen Coconut Vanilla Custard (page 257).

☑ **Allergy/Intolerance Substitutions:**
Tree nuts: In step 2, use vanilla extract instead of the almond extract. In step 5, replace the almond meal with an equal measure of pumpkin seed meal or sunflower seed meal (as tolerated; see page 72).

Eggs: Prepare in one bowl the equivalent of two eggs using the Rising Egg Replacer (page 74). In a second bowl, prepare the equivalent of one whole egg using the Non-rising Egg Replacer (page 76). In step 2, for the batter, leave out the eggs and add 5 T. (75 ml) of the Rising Egg Replacer (add 2 t. or 10 ml apple cider vinegar directly to the batter instead of to the egg replacer as specified in the Rising Egg Replacer recipe). In step 5, for the crumb topping, replace the egg white with 3 T. (45 ml) of the Non-Rising Egg Replacer.

☑ Reduced Sugar:

In step 1, leave out the sugar. In step 2, add 70 drops of clear, alcohol-free liquid stevia, ¼ cup (62 g) unsweetened apple sauce, ¼ t. (1 ml) lemon extract (in addition to the almond or vanilla extract included), and 1 t. (5 ml) apple cider vinegar (leave out this vinegar if using the Rising Egg Replacer since the replacer already includes vinegar). In step 5, for the crumb topping, leave out the sugar; add 50 drops of liquid stevia and an extra ½ t. (1.5 g) cinnamon (i.e., 1 t. or 3 g cinnamon total).

Batter Ingredients:
1½ c. gluten-free flour mix (195 g)
1 t. baking powder (5 g)
½ c. refined cane sugar (100 g)
2 large eggs
½ c. milk of choice (118 ml)
¼ c. pure olive oil (not extra virgin) or other neutral-flavored oil (59 ml)
1 T. almond or vanilla extract (15 ml)
1 cup fresh blueberries (140 g)

Crumb Topping Ingredients:
¾ c. almond meal (75 g)
½ c. refined cane sugar (100 g)
½ c. gluten-free flour mix (65 g)
½ t. cinnamon (1.5 g)
1 egg white
2 to 3 T. shortening or lard (18 to 27 g)

Preheat Oven: 350° F/177° C

Directions:

Step 1. For the batter, mix the 1½ cups (195 g) gluten-free flour mix, 1 t. (5 g) baking powder, and ½ cup (100 g) sugar together in a large mixing bowl.

Step 2. In a small bowl, whisk together the eggs, milk of choice, oil, and almond or vanilla extract. Add this mixture to the dry ingredients, mixing well with a rubber spatula to form a smooth batter.

Step 3. Blot the blueberries dry with a paper towel if they are wet. Gently fold the blueberries into the batter.

Step 4. Spray a square 8" x 8" (20 cm x 20 cm) pan with cooking oil. Pour the batter into the pan and spread it evenly with a rubber spatula.

Step 5. For the crumb topping, mix together (in a small mixing bowl) the almond meal, ½ cup (100 g) sugar, ½ cup (65 g) gluten-free flour mix, and cinnamon. Add the egg white and 2 T. (18 g) of shortening or lard; combine the ingredients with your hands till no lumps of shortening/lard can be seen. The crumb topping should be slightly sticky in texture. Test the crumbs by squeezing some in your hands; if large crumbs form and don't fall apart, the crumbs contain the correct amount of shortening/lard. If crumbs do not form, add one additional tablespoon (9 g) of shortening/lard, and mix into the crumb mixture; re-test the crumbs to see if they hold together when squeezed.

Step 6. Squeeze the topping mixture into pea-sized (or larger) crumbs with your hands as you sprinkle the crumbs on the top of the batter.

Step 7. Bake for about 35 to 40 minutes, until a toothpick inserted in the center of the cake comes out clean. Serve warm straight from the pan.

Nutritional content: Makes 9 servings (1 square piece (123 g) per serving). Each serving contains: Calories (370); Total Fat (15 g); Saturated Fat (3 g); Cholesterol (40 mg); Sodium (260 mg); Potassium (73 mg); Total Carbohydrate (54 g); Dietary Fiber (3 g); Sugars (25 g); Protein (6 g). Nutrient(s) of note (percent of Daily Value): Vitamin A 2%, Calcium 6%, Vitamin C 2%, Iron 6%

Blueberry Muffins:

Follow the recipe for Blueberry Crumb Cake as directed through Step 3. In step 4, fill lined muffin cups three-quarters full with the batter. Follow steps 5 and 6 as directed. Bake for 20 to 25 minutes, until a toothpick inserted in the center of the largest muffin comes out clean.

Peach Upside-down Cake

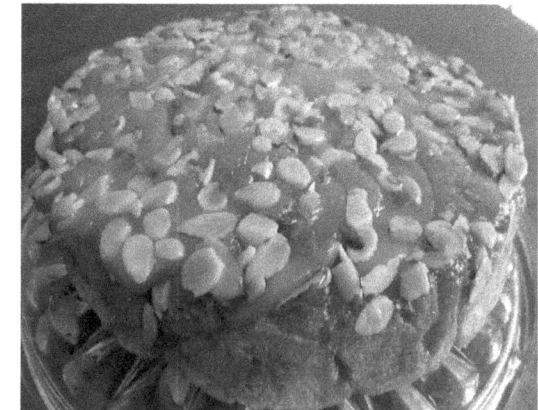

This is a moist and delicious cake with a rich caramelized almond and peach topping. If you use canned peaches instead of fresh, make sure to dab them with a paper towel to remove any excess liquid. Serve warm with some Frozen Coconut Vanilla Custard (page 257).

☑ Allergy/Intolerance Substitutions:

Tree nuts: In step 2, leave out the sliced almonds. In step 6, use vanilla extract instead of the almond extract.

Eggs: Prepare the equivalent of *one* egg using the Rising Egg Replacer (page 74). In step 6, leave out the eggs and add the egg replacer (be sure to add the apple cider vinegar as specified in the egg replacer recipe). This egg free version does not rise as well as the original; double the batter recipe for a higher cake.

☑ Reduced Sugar:

No suggestions given; this recipe does not work well without the sugar in the batter.

Topping Ingredients:
1 can of sliced peaches (15 oz. or 425 g) or 1 whole peach (not overly ripe), pitted and peeled
¼ c. sliced almonds (25 g)
½ c. lightly-packed brown sugar (72 g)
2 T. pure olive oil (not extra virgin) or other neutral-flavored oil (30 ml)

Batter Ingredients:
1½ c. gluten-free flour mix (195 g)
1 t. baking powder (5 g)
½ c. refined cane sugar (100 g)
2 large eggs
¾ c. milk of choice (177 ml)
¼ c. pure olive oil (not extra virgin) or other neutral-flavored oil (59 ml)
1 T. almond or vanilla extract (15 ml)

Preheat Oven: 350° F/177° C

Directions:
Step 1. Slice the peach into ¼-inch-thick segments (0.6 cm thick). Blot them dry with a paper towel to remove any excess moisture.

Step 2. For the topping, mix together in a small bowl the sliced almonds, brown sugar, and 2 T. (30 ml) olive oil (the mixture should be grainy in texture).

Step 3. Place a 10-inch-long (25-cm-long) piece of non-stick aluminum foil on a cutting board. Place an 8" (20 cm) round cake pan (bottom side down) on the foil. Use a pencil to trace the outline of the pan onto the foil, and then cut the foil on the line. Place the circle of foil (non-stick side facing up) in the bottom of the pan. Spray the foil and sides of the pan with cooking spray.

Step 4. Spread the topping mixture evenly on the foil in the bottom of the pan. Lay the peach slices (in a circular pattern) on top of the topping mixture. Set the pan aside.

Step 5. For the batter, mix the 1½ cups (195 g) gluten-free flour mix, baking powder, and ½ cup (100 g) sugar together in a large mixing bowl.

Step 6. In a medium-sized bowl, whisk together the eggs, milk of choice, oil, and almond or vanilla extract. Add this mixture to the dry ingredients; mix with a rubber spatula to form a smooth batter.

Step 7. Pour the batter evenly over the peaches in the baking pan (be careful to not move either the peaches or the topping as you pour). Carefully spread the batter into the corners of the pan with a rubber spatula and smooth the top. Gently shake the pan side to side to remove air pockets.

Step 8. Bake 35 to 40 minutes, until a toothpick inserted in the center of the cake comes out clean. Cool for 15 minutes. If the cake has risen too high in the middle, use a long, serrated bread knife to gently slice off a very thin layer from the middle of the cake to make it slightly flatter (this will prevent your cake from cracking when you turn it over).

Step 9. Carefully turn the pan upside down (with the foil still attached to the cake) onto a cake plate, and remove the pan. Gently peel off the aluminum foil; if any nuts or peaches are pulled off while removing the foil, simply put them back in place on the cake. Serve the cake warm or at room temperature.

Nutritional content: Makes 12 servings (1 slice (65 g) per serving; includes almonds). Each serving contains: Calories (200); Total Fat (9 g); Saturated Fat (1.5 g); Cholesterol (30 mg); Sodium (160 mg); Potassium (66 mg); Total Carbohydrate (28 g); Dietary Fiber (1 g); Sugars (13 g); Protein (2 g). Nutrient(s) of note (percent of Daily Value): Vitamin A 2%, Calcium 4%, Iron 4%

A Healthier Topping:

Skip step 2 completely. In step 4, drizzle the aluminum foil in the pan with ¼ cup (87 g) of honey and sprinkle with the sliced almonds. Lay the peach slices (in a circular pattern) on top of the honey and almonds. Pour the batter over the peaches in step 5 and bake as directed.

Chocolate Chip Cake

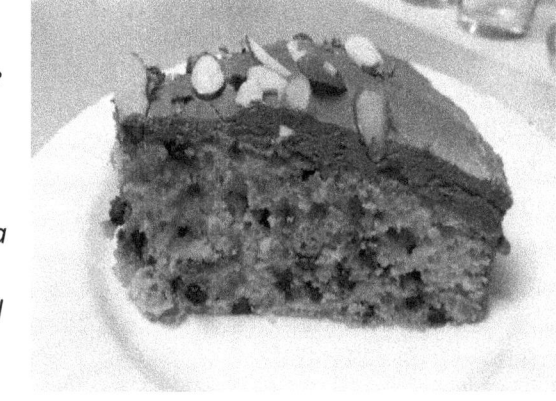

This single-layer cake is decadent! Frost with rich Chocolate Coconut Ganache or Frosting (page 249; the frosting is shown in the photo insert). This recipe is suitable for a birthday or other special event, and makes one 8-inch (20 cm) diameter cake layer; double the recipe for two layers or a 9" x 13" (23 cm x 33 cm) sheet pan.

☑ Allergy/Intolerance Substitutions:

Tree nuts: In step 2, replace the almond extract with vanilla extract.

Eggs: Prepare the equivalent of two eggs using the Rising Egg Replacer (page 74). In step 2, leave out the eggs and add the egg replacer (be sure to add the apple cider vinegar as specified in the egg replacer recipe). In step 4, if needed, smooth the top of the batter by brushing lightly with olive oil.

☑ Reduced Sugar:

In step 1, leave out the sugar and add 1 T. (4.5 g) coconut flour (if tolerated) to the dry ingredients. In step 2, add 75 drops of clear, alcohol-free liquid stevia and 1 t. (5 ml) apple cider vinegar (do not add this vinegar if using the

Rising Egg Replacer, as apple cider vinegar is already included in the egg replacer recipe). In step 3, use sugar-free GF-DF-SF chocolate or carob chips. In step 4, smooth the top of the batter with a rubber spatula; gently brush it with a pastry brush dipped in egg white or olive oil to smooth it completely. Bake as directed.

Batter Ingredients:
1½ c. gluten-free flour mix (195 g)
1 t. baking powder (5 g)
½ c. refined cane sugar (100 g)
2 large eggs
½ c. milk of choice (118 ml)
⅓ c. pure olive oil (not extra virgin) or other neutral-flavored oil (79 ml)
1 T. almond extract (15 ml)
½ c. GF-DF-SF chocolate chips (90 g)

Preheat Oven: 350° F/177° C

Directions:
Step 1. In a large mixing bowl, mix together the dry ingredients.

Step 2. In a small bowl, whisk together the eggs, milk of choice, oil, and almond extract. Add this mixture to the dry ingredients, mixing well with a rubber spatula to form a smooth batter.

Step 3. Stir in the chocolate chips.

Step 4. Spray an 8" x 8" (20 cm x 20 cm) square or 8" (20 cm) round pan with cooking oil. Pour the batter into the pan and spread it evenly with a rubber spatula.

Step 5. Bake for about 25 to 30 minutes, until a toothpick inserted in the center comes out clean. Remove the pan from the oven. Cool the cake for one hour before removing it from the pan; you can also leave the cake in the pan for serving if you wish.

Step 6. Cool the cake completely before frosting.

Nutritional content: Makes 9 servings (1 slice (76 g) per serving; frosting excluded). Each serving contains: Calories (240); Total Fat (11 g); Saturated Fat (2.5 g); Cholesterol (40 mg); Sodium (210 mg); Potassium (95 mg); Total Carbohydrate (35 g); Dietary Fiber (1 g); Sugars (14 g); Protein (3 g). Nutrient(s) of note (percent of Daily Value): Vitamin A 2%, Calcium 4%, Iron 6%

Fresh Strawberry Cake

The sweetness of the strawberries comes through in this cake, which I frequently make during strawberry season. To ensure the correct moisture content in the batter, be sure to measure the 1½ cups (220-230 g) of strawberries after they have been washed, dried, 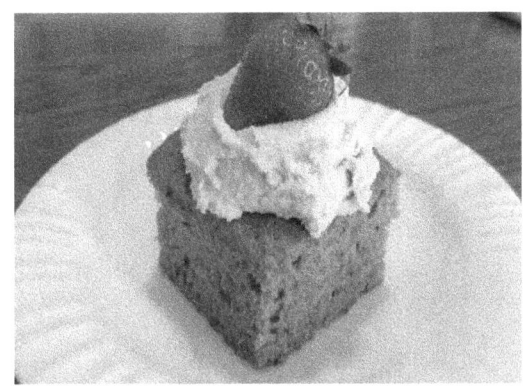 topped to remove the greens, and sliced in half. If your strawberries are large, cut them into quarters before measuring. For a cake that is pinker in color, add a little beet powder. For a stronger strawberry flavor, add 1 t. (5 ml) strawberry extract. This recipe makes one 8" x 8" (20 cm x 20 cm) square or one 8" or 9" (20 or 23 cm) diameter round cake layer; double the recipe for two layers. Serve with some fresh strawberries and the Cashew Coconut Cream Topping (shown in the photo insert; see page 245) or simply sprinkle with confectioner's sugar.

☑ Allergy/Intolerance Substitutions:

<u>Corn:</u> In step 6, either leave off the confectioner's sugar, or make your own with tapioca starch (see page 70).

<u>Eggs:</u> No suggestions given; this recipe does not work well with egg replacer.

☑ Reduced Sugar:
No suggestions given; this recipe does not work well without sugar.

Batter Ingredients:
1½ c. halved and quartered strawberries in ¾" to 1" (2 cm to 2.5 cm) chunks, tops removed (220 – 230 g)
¼ c. milk of choice (59 ml)
1½ c. gluten-free flour mix (195 g)
½ c. refined cane sugar (100 g)
1 t. baking powder (5 g)
2 large eggs
¼ c. pure olive oil (not extra virgin) or other neutral-flavored oil (59 ml)
1 T. vanilla extract (15 ml)

Preheat Oven: 350° F/177° C

Directions:
Step 1. Puree the 1½ cups (220-230 g) of halved strawberries in a blender with the milk of choice. Measure out 1 cup (237 ml) of the puree. If the puree is under 1 cup (237 ml), add a little extra milk of choice to bring it to 1 cup (237 ml).

Step 2. In a large mixing bowl, combine the gluten-free flour mix, sugar, and baking powder.

Step 3. In a small mixing bowl, whisk together the cup (237 ml) of pureed strawberries, eggs, oil, and vanilla extract. Add this mixture to the dry ingredients, mixing well with a rubber spatula till the batter is smooth.

Step 4. Spray an 8" x 8" (20 cm x 20 cm) pan, or 8" or 9" (20 cm or 23 cm) round cake pan with cooking oil. Pour the batter into the pan, and spread it out evenly with a rubber spatula. Gently shake the pan from side to side to level the batter out further.

Step 5. Bake for 30 to 35 minutes, until a toothpick inserted in the center of the cake comes out clean. Cool the cake for one hour, and then remove it from the pan.

Step 6. Cool completely to room temperature. Decorate the cake by either sprinkling with confectioner's sugar, or topping with sliced strawberries and Cashew-Coconut Cream (see page 245).

Nutritional content: Makes 9 servings (1 square piece (82 g) per serving; excludes toppings). Each serving contains: Calories (180); Total Fat (8 g); Saturated Fat (1.5 g); Cholesterol (40 mg); Sodium (180 mg); Potassium (79 mg); Total Carbohydrate (27 g); Dietary Fiber (1 g); Sugars (10 g); Protein (2 g). Nutrient(s) of note (percent of Daily Value): Vitamin A 2%, Calcium 2%, Vitamin C 25%, Iron 4%

Maple Berry Crunch

When it's berry season and you don't want to take the time to make a pie, make this recipe! It takes about 10 minutes to put together (not including the baking time) and tastes great. I make this with raspberries, blueberries, or blackberries—a mix of different types of berries works well, too! I also make this with sliced green apples instead of the berries. Serve with some Cashew-coconut Cream topping, Coconut Yogurt, or Frozen Coconut Vanilla Custard (see the last chapter for these recipes).

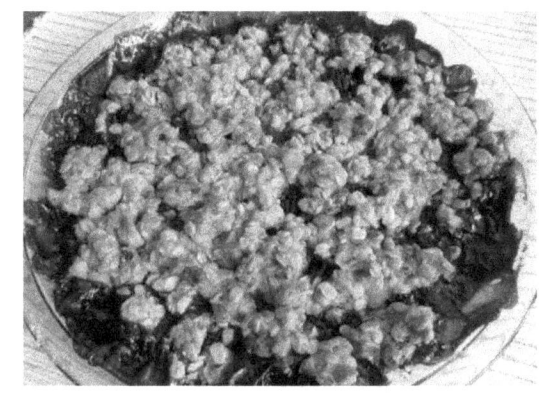

☑ **Allergy/Intolerance Substitutions:**
Tree nuts: In step 3, leave out the pecans.
Oats: In step 3, leave out the oats; add ½ cup (50 g) almond meal, dry quinoa flakes, pumpkin seed meal, or sunflower seed meal (as tolerated).

☑ **Reduced Sugar:**
In step 2, leave out the maple syrup; add ¼ cup (62 g) unsweetened applesauce that has been mixed with 40 drops of alcohol-free liquid stevia. In step 4, replace the maple syrup in the crumb topping with 50 drops of clear, alcohol-free liquid stevia.

Filling Ingredients:
2 c. fresh berries (blueberries, raspberries, or blackberries), washed and dried (280 g)
1 T. tapioca starch (8 g)
¼ c. maple syrup (59 ml)
1 t. vanilla extract (5 ml)

Crumb Topping Ingredients:
½ c. gluten-free flour mix (65 g)
¾ c. certified GF rolled oats (75 g)
⅓ c. chopped pecans (34 g)
½ t. cinnamon (1.5 g)
¼ c. shortening or lard (36 g)
¼ c. maple syrup (59 ml)

Preheat Oven: 350° F/177° C

Directions:
Step 1. For the filling, mix the berries with the tapioca starch in a pie pan till the berries are well-coated with the starch.

Step 2. In a small bowl, combine the ¼ cup (59 ml) of maple syrup with the vanilla extract. Drizzle the syrup mixture over the top of the berries. Gently stir the berries till they are coated with the syrup. Spread the berries evenly in the pie pan. Set the pan aside.

Step 3. For the crumb topping, combine the gluten-free flour mix, rolled oats, pecans, and cinnamon in a small mixing bowl.

Step 4. Add the shortening/lard and ¼ cup (59 ml) maple syrup to the crumb topping ingredients; combine well with your hands, till no lumps of shortening/lard remain (the mixture will be soft and sticky).

Step 5. Sprinkle clumps of the topping on top of the berry mixture in the pie pan, leaving small spaces where the berries show through.

Step 6. Place the pie pan in the oven. Bake for 35 minutes, or until the berry mixture is bubbling and the topping is a light golden brown. Cool for ten minutes before serving.

Nutritional content: Makes 8 servings (one large scoop (88 g) per serving; includes blueberries). Each serving contains: Calories (231); Total Fat (11 g); Saturated Fat (3.5 g); Cholesterol (0 mg); Sodium (48 mg); Potassium (97 mg); Total Carbohydrate (34 g); Dietary Fiber (3 g); Sugars (18 g); Protein (2 g). Nutrient(s) of note (percent of Daily Value): Calcium 4%, Vitamin C 6%, Iron 6%

Biscuit, Pizza, and Pie Doughs

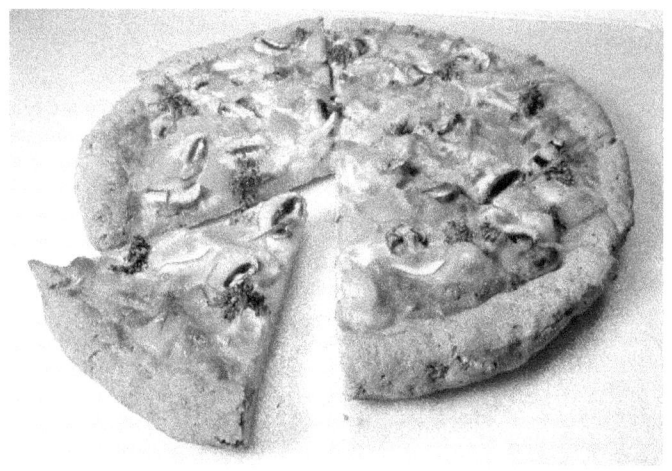

Basic Dinner Biscuits

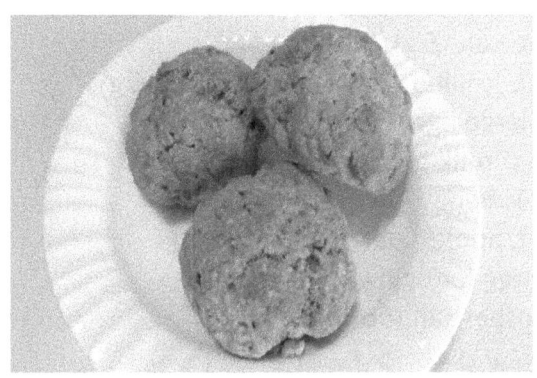

This simple and hearty biscuit goes well with any meal. It's best when served warm. Makes about 8 biscuits.

☑ Allergy/Intolerance Substitutions:
Eggs: Prepare the egg replacer equivalent of one egg using either the Non-rising Egg Replacer (page 76) or the Chia Seed Egg Replacer (page 74). In step 3, replace the egg with the egg replacer. In step 5, brush the dough with olive oil or other cooking oil instead of the egg wash.

☑ Reduced Sugar:
In step 3, replace the honey in the dough with 10 drops of clear, alcohol-free liquid stevia.

Dough Ingredients:
1⅔ c. gluten-free flour mix (224 g)
⅓ c. arrowroot or tapioca starch (44 g)
1½ t. baking powder (7.5 g)
1 t. salt (6 g)
¼ c. chilled shortening or lard (36 g)
1 large egg
⅔ c. milk of choice (158 ml)
2 T. honey (44 g)
1 t. apple cider vinegar (5 ml)
1 egg for egg wash (optional)
Kosher salt (optional)

Preheat Oven: 350° F/177° C

Directions:
Step 1. In a large mixing bowl, mix together the gluten-free flour mix, arrowroot or tapioca starch, baking powder, and salt.

Step 2. Cut the shortening or lard into the dry ingredients with a pastry cutter till the shortening is in pea-sized pieces and well-coated with the flour mixture.

Step 3. In a small mixing bowl, whisk together one egg, the milk of choice, honey, and apple cider vinegar; pour into the flour mixture. Using a rubber spatula, combine until a thick, sticky dough forms (do not over-mix).

Step 4. Spray a cookie sheet with cooking oil. Using a large spoon, scoop out approximately ⅓ cup (82 g) of dough. Roll the dough gently in your hands to form a ball that is about two inches (5 cm) in diameter. Place the ball on the cookie sheet, and flatten the top slightly with your fingertips. Repeat with the remainder of the dough, spacing the balls of dough about two inches (5 cm) apart on the cookie sheet.

Step 5. Brush the dough balls with an "egg wash" made from one whisked egg (optional). Gently smooth each dough ball with the brush as you apply the egg wash.

Step 6. Sprinkle each dough ball with a pinch of coarse kosher salt (optional).

Step 7. Bake for 15 to 17 minutes, till the tops of the biscuits turn golden brown. Serve hot from the oven.

Nutritional content: Makes 8 servings (1 biscuit (75 g) per serving; excludes egg wash and Kosher salt). Each serving contains: Calories (210); Total Fat (8 g); Saturated Fat (3 g); Cholesterol (25 mg); Sodium (570 mg); Potassium (48 mg); Total Carbohydrate (35 g); Dietary Fiber (1 g); Sugars (5 g); Protein (2 g). Nutrient(s) of note (percent of Daily Value): Vitamin A 2%, Calcium 4%, Iron 4%

Rosemary-Garlic Biscuits

These biscuits have a wonderful garlic and rosemary flavor. Other herbs can be used in place of the rosemary if desired. Best when served warm. Makes about 8 biscuits.

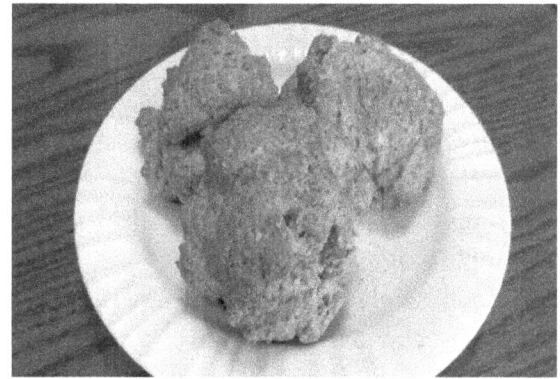

☑ **Allergy/Intolerance Substitutions:**
Eggs: Prepare the egg replacer equivalent of one egg using either the Non-rising Egg Replacer (page 76) or the Chia Seed Egg Replacer (page 74). In step 5, replace the egg with the egg replacer. In step 8, brush the dough with olive oil or other cooking oil instead of the egg wash.

☑ **Reduced Sugar:**
In step 5, replace the honey in the dough with 10 drops of clear, alcohol-free liquid stevia.

Dough Ingredients:
1 head of garlic
1⅔ c. gluten-free flour mix (224 g)
⅓ c. arrowroot or tapioca starch (44 g)
1½ t. baking powder (7.5 g)
1 T. garlic powder (9 g)
1 t. salt (6 g)
¼ c. chilled shortening or lard (36 g)
1 large egg
⅔ c. milk of choice (158 ml)
2 T. honey (44 g)
1 t. apple cider vinegar (5 ml)
1 T. fresh, finely-minced rosemary (6 g)
1 egg for egg wash (optional)
Kosher salt

Preheat Oven: 350° F/ 177° C

Directions:
Step 1. Slice the top off a head of garlic (you should be able to see the tops of the cloves). Place in a pan root-side down and drizzle with a little olive oil. Roast in the oven till the cloves are soft when pinched and golden in color (30 to 45 minutes).

Step 2. Squeeze four large cloves of garlic out of their husks, and roughly chop them. (Note: Store the unused, peeled garlic cloves in the refrigerator in a container filled with olive oil for future recipes).

Step 3. In a large mixing bowl, mix together the dry ingredients.

Step 4. Cut the shortening or lard into the dry ingredients with a pastry cutter till the shortening/lard is in pea-sized pieces and well-coated with the flour mixture.

Step 5. In a small mixing bowl, whisk together one egg, the milk of choice, honey, and apple cider vinegar; pour into the flour mixture. Using a rubber spatula, combine until a thick, sticky dough forms (do not over-mix).

Step 6. Mix in the chopped garlic and minced rosemary.

Step 7. Spray a cookie sheet with cooking oil. Using a large spoon, scoop out approximately ⅓ cup (82 g) of dough. Roll the dough gently in your hands to form a ball that is about 2 inches (5 cm) in diameter. Place the ball on the cookie sheet, and flatten the top slightly with your fingertips. Repeat with the remainder of the dough, spacing the balls of dough about two inches (5 cm) apart on the cookie sheet.

Step 8. Brush the top of the biscuits with an "egg wash" made from one whisked egg (optional). Sprinkle the biscuits with a pinch of Kosher salt (optional).

Step 9. Bake for 15 to 17 minutes, till the edges of the biscuits start to brown and the tops become golden. Serve hot from the oven.

Nutritional content: Makes 8 servings (1 biscuit (78 g) per serving; excludes egg wash and Kosher salt). Each serving contains: Calories (220); Total Fat (8 g); Saturated Fat (3 g); Cholesterol (25 mg); Sodium (570 mg); Potassium (68 mg); Total Carbohydrate (36 g); Dietary Fiber (2 g); Sugars (5 g); Protein (2 g). Nutrient(s) of note (percent of Daily Value): Vitamin A 2%, Calcium 4%, Iron 4%

Cranberry Orange Scones

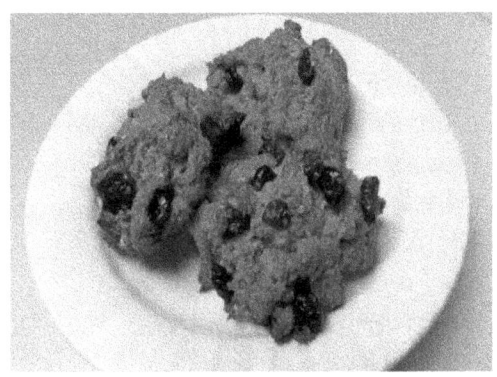

Scrumptious as a dessert or snack, these scones can also be served with dinner. Makes about 6 scones.

☑ Allergy/Intolerance Substitutions:
Eggs: Prepare the egg replacer equivalent of one egg using the Non-rising Egg Replacer (page 76). In step 3, add the egg replacer, and reduce the amount of milk of choice added to 3 T. (45 ml). In step 6, leave off the egg wash.

☑ Reduced Sugar:
In step 3, replace the honey in the dough with 40 to 45 drops of clear, alcohol-free liquid stevia. Add an extra ⅓ cup (79 ml) of milk of choice (i.e., ⅔ cup or 158 ml total). In step 4, use only unsweetened dried cranberries. In step 6, do not sprinkle with coarse sugar.

Dough Ingredients:
1½ c. gluten-free flour mix (195 g)
1 t. baking powder (5 g)
¼ c. chilled shortening or lard (36 g)
1 large egg
⅓ c. milk of choice (79 ml)
¼ c. honey (87 g)
1 T. orange extract (15 ml)
1 T. fresh orange zest (6 g)
½ c. dried cranberries (80 g)
1 egg for egg wash (optional)
Coarse sugar (optional)

Preheat Oven: 400° F/204° C

Directions:
Step 1. In a large mixing bowl, combine the gluten-free flour mix and baking powder.

Step 2. Cut the shortening or lard into the dry ingredients with a pastry cutter till the shortening is in pea-sized pieces and well-coated with the flour mixture.

Step 3. In a small bowl, whisk together the egg, milk of choice, honey, and orange extract and zest. Add this mixture to the dry ingredients, mixing with a rubber spatula or your hands till a thick and sticky dough forms (do not over-mix).

Step 4. Fold in the dried cranberries.

Step 5. Spray a cookie sheet with cooking oil. Drop heaping Tablespoons (approximately ¼ cup or 65 g) of the dough onto the cookie sheet. Gently shape the edges of the scones into an oval shape. Avoid rolling the dough in your hands as this will make the scones denser in texture. (Note: how these scones look going into the oven is how they will look after baking).

Step 6. Brush the top of the scones with an "egg wash" made from one whisked egg (optional). Sprinkle the scones with a pinch of coarse or raw sugar (optional).

Step 7. Bake for 12 to 15 minutes, till the edges of the scones start to brown and the tops become golden. Serve warm.

Nutritional content: Makes 6 servings (1 scone (95 g) per serving; excludes egg wash and coarse sugar). Each serving contains: Calories (300); Total Fat (10 g); Saturated Fat (4.5 g); Cholesterol (30 mg); Sodium (290 mg); Potassium (61 mg); Total Carbohydrate (50 g); Dietary Fiber (2 g); Sugars (18 g); Protein (3 g). Nutrient(s) of note (percent of Daily Value): Vitamin A 2%, Calcium 4%, Vitamin C 2%, Iron 4%

Blueberry Scones

These scones bake quickly and disappear just as quickly.
This recipe does not work well with frozen blueberries, or frozen and thawed blueberries; use fresh blueberries only. Makes about 6 scones.

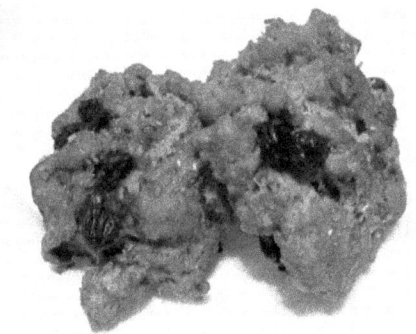

☑ **Allergy/Intolerance Substitutions:**
Eggs: Prepare the egg replacer equivalent of one egg using the Non-rising Egg Replacer (page 76). In step 3, add the egg replacer, and reduce the amount of milk of choice added to 3 T. (45 ml). In step 6, leave off the egg wash.

☑ **Reduced Sugar:**
In step 3, replace the honey in the dough with 40 to 45 drops of clear, alcohol-free liquid stevia. Add an extra ⅓ cup (79 ml) of milk of choice (i.e., ⅔ cup or 158 ml total). In step 6, do not sprinkle with coarse sugar.

Dough Ingredients:
1½ c. gluten-free flour mix (195 g)
1 t. baking powder (5 g)
¼ c. chilled shortening or lard (36 g)
1 large egg
⅓ c. milk of choice (79 ml)
¼ c. honey (87 g)
1 T. vanilla extract (15 ml)
½ c. fresh blueberries (70 g)
1 egg for egg wash (optional)
Coarse sugar (optional)

Preheat Oven: 400° F/204° C

Directions:
Step 1. In a large mixing bowl, combine the gluten-free flour mix and baking powder.

Step 2. Cut the shortening or lard into the dry ingredients with a pastry cutter till the shortening is in pea-sized pieces and well-coated with the flour mixture.

Step 3. In a small mixing bowl, whisk together the egg, milk of choice, honey, and vanilla extract. Add this mixture to the dry ingredients, mixing with a rubber spatula or your hands till a thick and sticky dough forms (do not over-mix).

Step 4. Blot the blueberries dry with a paper towel if they are wet. Gently fold them into the dough.

Step 5. Spray a cookie sheet with cooking oil. Drop heaping Tablespoons (approximately ¼ cup or 65 g) of the dough onto the cookie sheet. Gently shape the edges of the scones into an oval shape. Avoid rolling the dough in your hands as this will make the scones denser in texture. (Note: how these scones look going into the oven is how they will look after baking).

Step 6. Brush the top of the scones with an "egg wash" made from one whisked egg (optional). Sprinkle the scones with a pinch of coarse or raw sugar (optional).

Step 7. Bake for 12 to 15 minutes, till the edges of the scones start to brown and the tops become slightly golden. Serve warm.

Nutritional content: Makes 6 servings (1 scone (96 g) per serving; excludes egg wash and coarse sugar). Each serving contains: Calories (270); Total Fat (10 g); Saturated Fat (4.5 g); Cholesterol (30 mg); Sodium (290 mg); Potassium (67 mg); Total Carbohydrate (44 g); Dietary Fiber (2 g); Sugars (13 g); Protein (3 g). Nutrient(s) of note (percent of Daily Value): Vitamin A 2%, Calcium 4%, Vitamin C 2%, Iron 4%

Pizza Dough

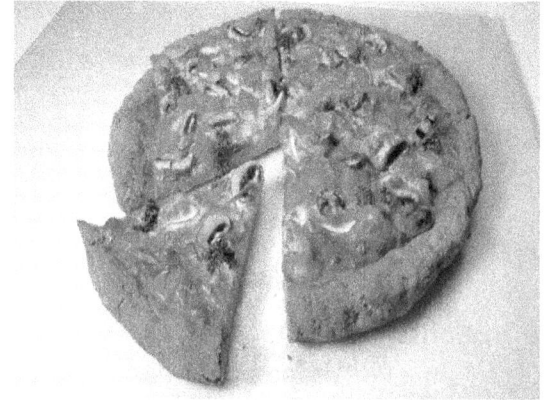

This recipe makes either one thick-crust pizza or two thin-crust pizzas. The almond meal sweetens the taste of the gluten-free flours, and makes the crust crisp. Make sure that rapid rise yeast is used (active dry yeast does not work as well with this recipe).

☑ **Allergy/Intolerance Substitutions:**
Tree nuts: In step 1, replace the almond meal with pumpkin seed meal or sunflower seed meal.
Rice: In step 1, replace the sweet rice flour with tapioca starch.
Eggs: Prepare the egg replacer equivalent of one egg using the Rising Egg Replacer (page 74). In step 2, replace the egg with the egg replacer (be sure to add the apple cider vinegar as directed in the egg replacer recipe).
Yeast: Avoid this recipe.

☑ **Reduced Sugar:**
No suggestions given; the yeast will not activate without the honey.

Dough Ingredients:
2 c. gluten-free flour mix (260 g)
¼ c. almond meal (25 g)
½ c. sweet rice flour (60 g)
1 t. salt (6 g)
1 t. garlic powder (optional) (3 g)
2¼ t. (one packet) rapid rise yeast (8.5 g)
1 large egg
1 T. honey (22 g)
1 c. hot tap water (237 ml)

Preheat Oven: lowest setting (warm)

Directions:
Step 1. In a large food processor or mixing bowl, mix together the dry ingredients, including the yeast.

Step 2. In a small mixing bowl, whisk together the egg, honey, and hot tap water till the mixture is slightly frothy.

Step 3. Add the egg-water mixture to the dry ingredients and combine well with the food processor or your hands till a smooth, thick, sticky dough forms.

Step 4. *If using a pizza pan:* For one thick crust pizza, spray a pizza pan with cooking spray and place all of the dough on the pan. Spray the top of the dough with cooking spray, and cover with plastic wrap. Using the palm of your hand (on top of the plastic-wrap-covered dough), spread the dough evenly till it is about ½ inch (approximately 1 cm) thick; leave a thicker crust around the edge of the pan.

For two thin crust pizzas, spray two pizza pans and place half of the dough on each pan. Spray the top of the dough with cooking spray, and cover with plastic wrap. Use a rolling pin on top of the plastic-wrap-covered dough to spread the dough to a thickness of about ¼ inch (0.6 cm).

If using a pizza stone: For one thick crust pizza, line a flat, moveable, and heat resistant surface (e.g., a rimless cookie sheet) with parchment paper; place the dough on top of the parchment. Spray the top of the dough with cooking spray, and cover with plastic wrap. Using the palm of your hand (on top of the plastic-wrap-covered dough), spread the dough evenly on the parchment paper to form a circle that is about 12 inches (30 cm) in diameter and about ½ inch (1 cm) thick; leave a thicker crust around the edge. (Note: avoid using a pizza stone for thin crust pizzas; they do not roll out well on parchment paper.)

Step 5. Turn off the oven. Leaving the plastic wrap on top of the dough, place the pan(s) in the warmed oven. Let the dough rise for 10 minutes.

Step 6. Remove the pan(s) from the oven. If using a pizza stone, place the stone in the oven. Pre-heat the oven to 500° F/260° C.

Step 7. Remove the plastic wrap from the top of the dough. Spray or brush the crust(s) with olive oil (optional).

Step 8. *If using a pizza pan:* Place the pizza pan(s) in the oven and reduce the oven temperature to 415° F/213° C. For the thin crust pizza, bake for 5 minutes; for the thick crust, bake for 8 to 10 minutes, until the top of the dough begins to look dry. Remove the crust(s) from the oven and top with tomato sauce or pesto, GF-DF-SF cheese, sautéed vegetables, or other toppings. Bake for an additional 15 to 25 minutes till the center of the pizza no longer appears doughy, and the cheese (if used) becomes a golden brown.

If using a pizza stone: Top the *raw* dough with tomato sauce or pesto, GF-DF-SF cheese, sautéed vegetables, or other toppings. Slide the parchment paper and dough together onto the hot pizza stone in the oven. Reduce the oven temperature to 415° F/213° C. Bake for 20 to 30 minutes till the center of the pizza no longer appears doughy, and the cheese (if used) becomes a golden brown.

Step 9. Remove the pizza(s) from the oven. Cool for five minutes before serving.

Nutritional content: Makes 8 servings (1 thick slice (91 g) per serving; excludes toppings). Each serving contains: Calories (200); Total Fat (3 g); Saturated Fat (0 g); Cholesterol (25 mg); Sodium (490 mg); Potassium (59 mg); Total Carbohydrate (41 g); Dietary Fiber (2 g); Sugars (2 g); Protein (4 g). Nutrient(s) of note (percent of Daily Value): Calcium 2%, Iron 6%

Single-crust Pie Dough

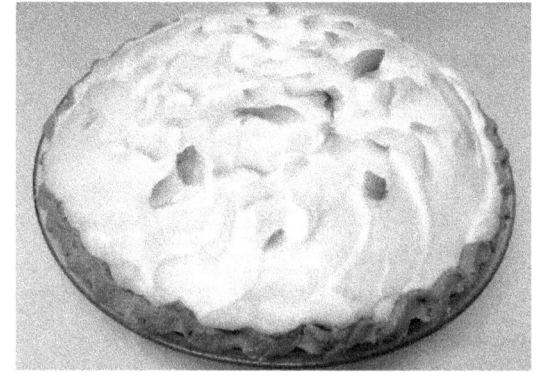

*T*his pie dough comes out flaky and golden. In order to make the dough mild in flavor and flexible, additional flours and starches are added. Wine or vodka can be used in this dough; the alcohol burns off during the baking process, leaving a crisp crust and no residual alcohol. For a light-colored crust, use a sweet white wine such as a pinot grigio; for a slightly darker crust (shown in the photo), a red wine such as a sweet Marsala works well; for an extra flaky and crisp crust, use an unflavored, gluten-free vodka; for those who cannot use alcohol, use water instead. Be sure to measure the liquids used in this recipe carefully. As long as a non-dairy shortening is used, you will most likely not need to cover the crust with aluminum foil to prevent it from burning. This recipe can be easily made in a large food processor.

☑ **Allergy/Intolerance Substitutions:**
Tree nuts: In step 1, replace the almond meal with an equivalent measure of pumpkin seed meal or sunflower seed meal (see page 72).
Eggs: Prepare the equivalent of one whole egg using the Non-rising Egg Replacer (page 76). In step 3, replace the

egg yolk with 2 T. (30 ml) of the egg replacer (discard the remaining egg replacer). If the dough is not adequately pliable after kneading, add an extra Tablespoon (15 ml) of wine, vodka, or water. In step 8, do not use an egg wash on the dough.

☑ Reduced Sugar:
In step 1, leave out the sugar. In step 3, add 10 drops of clear, alcohol-free liquid stevia (optional). Use water in place of the wine or vodka.

Dough Ingredients:
¾ c. gluten-free flour mix (96 g)
½ c. arrowroot or tapioca starch (60 g)
¼ c. almond meal (25 g)
¼ c. fava or garbanzo bean flour (26 g)
1 T. refined cane sugar (12 g)
⅛ t. salt (0.7 g)
¼ c. shortening or lard (36 g)
1 large egg yolk
¼ c. sweet red or white wine, unflavored GF vodka, or water (59 ml), plus extra for moistening if needed
1 egg white for egg wash (optional)

Preheat Oven: 350° F/177° C

Directions:
Step 1. Mix together the dry ingredients in a large mixing bowl or the bowl of a large food processor.

Step 2. Cut the shortening/lard into the dry ingredients with a pastry cutter or by pulsing in a food processor, until pea-sized pieces of flour-coated dough are formed (the dough will appear very crumbly and loose at this stage).

Step 3. In a small mixing bowl, whisk together the one egg yolk (set the egg white aside to use in step 8) and ¼ cup (59 ml) of the wine, vodka, or water. Pour into the dry ingredients. Mix well with your hands or with the food processor till the dough pulls together into a ball that is uniform in texture and easy to knead. If the dough is slightly dry and crumbly, add one extra teaspoon (5 ml) of wine, vodka, or water. Remove the dough from the food processor. Knead the dough by hand for an additional minute till it is smooth in texture.

Step 4. Form the dough into a ball and wrap it in wax paper. Let the wrapped dough rest at room temperature for 30 minutes (if the room temperature is above 70° F/ 21° C, place in a cool location (but not the refrigerator)).

Step 5. Roll out the dough between two sheets of plastic wrap till it is roughly 12 inches (30 cm) in diameter and ¼-inch (0.6 cm) thick. If the top sheet of plastic wrap gets stuck under the dough as you roll, simply pull it out from underneath the dough and continue rolling. (Note: It is okay if one-inch-long (2.5-cm-long) cracks form along the edge of the dough as you roll it out. If more extensive cracks appear in the dough, knead an additional teaspoon (5 ml) of wine, vodka, or water into the dough.)

Step 6. Gently remove the top piece of plastic wrap. Pick up the sheet of dough (with the remaining piece of plastic wrap attached underneath) and gently turn it over into an 8- or 9-inch (20- or 23-cm) pie pan (plastic-wrap side facing up); gently press the dough into the pie pan. Peel off the remaining sheet of plastic wrap. If part of the edge of your pie pan is not covered with dough, simply take a piece of leftover dough and pinch it into place till you can no longer see where the new piece was added; pinch together any cracks along the edge as well.

Step 7. If the edge of the dough extends past the rim of the pie pan, fold the edge of the dough under itself. Gently pinch the edge of the dough till it is roughly the same thickness around the entire edge. Flute the edge of the dough by crimping with a fork, or pinching as shown in the photo. Prick the dough on the bottom of the pan with a fork to prevent air bubbles from forming during the baking process.

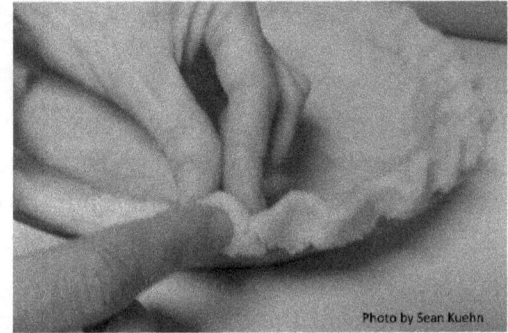

Step 8. Make an "egg wash" by whisking the egg white; brush the edge of the pie crust gently with the egg wash (this step is optional but will give your pie crust a deep golden, glossy color).

Step 9. *For a pie with a baked filling:* Bake the empty crust for 10 minutes at 350° F/177° C. Remove from the oven. Pour in the desired filling and bake according to the filling recipe.

For a pie with an unbaked filling: Place a foil-wrapped packet of dry beans or pie weights in the center of the pie crust, keeping the packet away from the crimped edge of the crust. (Note: The packet of beans/weights will prevent air bubbles from forming in your crust during the baking process. To make the packet, pour about 1 cup (220 g) of beans or pie weights onto a 12-inch-square (30-cm-square) sheet of aluminum foil; fold the foil over and crimp the edges to seal.) Bake the pie crust (with the packet of beans/weights in place) for 20 to 25 minutes at 350° F/177° C, or until the dough no longer looks raw and is golden in color. Take the crust out of the oven and remove the packet of beans/weights. Cool the pie crust and follow your recipe of choice for the filling.

Nutritional content: Makes 8 servings (1 slice (52 g) per serving; excludes pie filling). Each serving contains: Calories (200); Total Fat (11 g); Saturated Fat (4 g); Cholesterol (80 mg); Sodium (110 mg); Potassium (18 mg); Total Carbohydrate (23 g); Dietary Fiber (2 g); Sugars (2 g); Protein (3 g). Nutrient(s) of note (percent of Daily Value): Vitamin A 2%, Calcium 2%, Iron 4%

Blueberry Custard Pie Filling:

Make this delicious recipe the day before it is to be served to allow it time to thicken. Prepare a pie shell for a baked filling. Make the Frozen Coconut Vanilla Custard recipe on page 257, but modify it as follows: In step 6, as you heat the custard, gradually add ¼ cup (30 g) tapioca starch to the custard; mix constantly to prevent any lumps of starch from forming. After the custard has reached an adequate thickness and temperature (see the custard recipe for details), cool the custard to room temperature (do not freeze). Strain the custard through a fine mesh metal sieve to remove any lumps. Wash and blot dry 2 cups (280 g) fresh blueberries (frozen and thawed blueberries can also be used) and place in a mixing bowl. Sprinkle 2 T. (15 g) of tapioca starch over the blueberries; gently mix to coat the blueberries. Fill the baked pie crust with the blueberries, spreading them evenly in the crust. Pour the custard over the blueberries, filling the crust to slightly below the edge. Bake for 55 to 70 minutes at 350° F/177° C till the top of the filling bubbles slightly and turns golden brown. If the pie crust begins to brown too much because of the long baking time, cover its edge with aluminum foil. Remove the pie from the oven and cool at room temperature for 1 hour. Refrigerate overnight before serving.

Double-crust Pie Dough

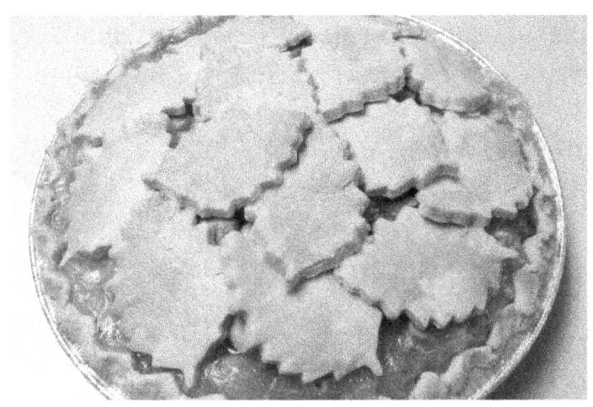

Double-crust gluten-free pies take a little more effort to prepare than single crust because the top crust can crack if not placed carefully on the filling. As with the single-crust recipe, use either a sweet white wine such as a pinot grigio for a light-colored crust, or a red wine such as a sweet Marsala for a slightly darker crust; for a crisper and flakier crust, use an unflavored, gluten-free vodka; for those who cannot use alcohol, use water instead. For a sealed pie, I recommend using water since all the alcohol in the bottom crust does not always burn off completely; the vodka in particular can leave a bitter aftertaste if it does not burn off. If you wish to use the wine or vodka, follow the Faux Double-crust Pie recipe (shown in the photo insert) on page 200 instead. This dough can be easily made in a large food processor.

☑ **Allergy/Intolerance Substitutions:**
Tree nuts: In step 1, replace the almond meal with an equivalent measure of pumpkin seed meal or sunflower seed meal (see page 72).
Eggs: Prepare the equivalent of one whole egg using the Non-rising Egg Replacer (page 76). In step 3, replace the

two egg yolks with all of the egg replacer. If the dough is not adequately pliable, add an extra tablespoon (15 ml) of wine, vodka, or water. In step 12, do not use an egg wash.

☑ Reduced Sugar:
In step 1, leave out the sugar. In step 3, add 15 drops of clear, alcohol-free liquid stevia (optional). Use water in place of the wine or vodka.

Dough Ingredients:
1½ c. gluten-free flour mix (195 g)
1 c. arrowroot or tapioca starch (120 g)
½ c. almond meal (50 g)
½ c. fava or garbanzo bean flour (52 g)
2 T. refined cane sugar (25 g)
¼ t. salt (1.5 g)
⅔ c. shortening or lard (100 g)
2 large egg yolks
½ c. sweet red or white wine, unflavored GF vodka, or water (118 ml), plus extra for moistening if needed
1 egg white for egg wash (optional)

Preheat Oven: Follow the baking instructions for your filling recipe.

Directions:
Step 1. Mix the dry ingredients together in a large mixing bowl or the bowl of a large food processor.

Step 2. Cut the shortening/lard into the dry ingredients with a pastry cutter or by pulsing in the food processor, until pea-sized pieces of flour-coated dough are formed (the dough will appear very crumbly and loose at this stage).

Step 3. In a small mixing bowl, whisk together the two egg yolks (set the egg whites aside to use in step 12) and ½ cup (118 ml) of the wine, vodka, or water. Pour into the dry ingredients. Mix well with your hands or with the food processor till the dough pulls together into a ball that is uniform in texture and moderately easy to knead. If the dough is slightly dry and crumbly, mix in one to two extra teaspoons (5 to 10 ml) of wine, vodka, or water. Knead the dough by hand for an additional minute till it is smooth in texture.

Step 4. Form the dough into a ball and wrap it in wax paper. Let the wrapped dough rest at room temperature for 30 minutes (if the room temperature is above 70° F/ 21° C, place it in a cool location (but not the refrigerator)).

Step 5. Divide the dough roughly in half, with one half slightly larger than the other. Roll out the larger half between two sheets of plastic wrap till it is roughly 12 inches (30 cm) in diameter and ¼-inch (0.6 cm) thick. If the top sheet of plastic wrap gets stuck under the dough as you roll, simply pull it out from underneath the dough and continue rolling. (Note: It is okay if one-inch-long (2.5-cm-long) cracks form along the edge of the dough as you roll it out; if more extensive cracks appear in the dough, knead an additional teaspoon (5 ml) of wine, vodka, or water into the dough.)

Step 6. Gently remove the top piece of plastic wrap. Pick up the sheet of dough (with the remaining sheet of plastic wrap attached underneath) and gently turn it over into an 8- or 9-inch (20- or 23-cm) pie pan (plastic-wrap side facing up); gently press the dough into the pie pan. Peel off the remaining sheet of plastic wrap.

Step 7. With a knife, slice off any dough that is hanging over the edge of the pan. If part of the edge of your pie pan is not covered with dough, simply take a piece of leftover dough and push it into place till you can no longer see where the new piece was added; pinch together any cracks along the edge as well. Prick the bottom of the dough with a fork to prevent air bubbles from forming in the crust during the baking process.

Step 8. Pour the filling of your choice into the dough-lined pie plate. Smooth the top of the filling, as bumps in the filling could crack the upper crust of dough when it is placed on top.

Step 9. Roll out a second sheet of dough between two new sheets of plastic wrap until it is roughly 11 inches (28 cm) in diameter and ¼-inch (0.6 cm) thick. If any cracks appear along the edge of the dough, peel back the top sheet of plastic wrap near the cracks, leaving most of the plastic wrap in place. Repair any cracks in the dough by pinching the cracks together, or by adding some dough to large cracks and pushing the dough into place. Lay the plastic wrap back over the dough, and gently roll over the repairs with a rolling pin till the dough is smooth.

Step 10. Peel off the top layer of plastic wrap. Gently flip the dough over and place it on top of the pie filling (the remaining sheet of plastic wrap should now be facing up). Be very careful when placing the top sheet of dough on the filling as you won't be able to move the dough once it is in place without cracking it. Gently peel off the remaining plastic wrap.

Step 11. Remove any dough hanging over the edge of the pan with a knife. Use your fingers to carefully pinch the top and bottom layers of dough together along the edge of the pan. Flute or crimp the edge. Cut a few steam vents into the top of the pie.

Step 12. Make an "egg wash" by whisking the egg whites; brush the pie crust gently with the egg wash (this step is optional but will give your pie crust a deep golden, glossy color). Depending on the shortening used, you probably will not need to cover the edge of the pie with aluminum foil to prevent the edge from burning (note: you usually only need to cover pies made with wheat flour or butter, but check your pie as it bakes just to be sure that it does not become too dark). Bake per the filling recipe instructions.

Nutritional content: Makes 8 servings (1 slice (103 g) per serving; excludes pie filling). Each serving contains: Calories (420); Total Fat (24 g); Saturated Fat (9 g); Cholesterol (110 mg); Sodium (220 mg); Potassium (31 mg); Total Carbohydrate (46 g); Dietary Fiber (4 g); Sugars (3 g); Protein (6 g). Nutrient(s) of note (percent of Daily Value): Vitamin A 2%, Calcium 4%, Iron 8%

Faux Double-Crust Pie:

Follow the original pie dough recipe through Step 7. Flute the edge of the bottom pie crust and bake at 350° F/177° C for 10 minutes. Remove the pie crust from the oven and fill with your filling of choice (only use a filling that can be baked). Roll out the remaining dough between two sheets of plastic wrap till it is ¼-inch (0.6 cm) thick. Remove the top sheet of plastic wrap. Use a small cookie cutter to cut out shapes such as stars or flowers. Peel one shape off the lower sheet of plastic wrap and place it on top of the pie filling; repeat for the other shapes, overlapping the shapes as desired. For drier fillings (such as sliced apples), cover as much of the filling as possible with the dough shapes; for juicier fillings (such as blueberries), larger gaps can be kept between the dough shapes. Brush the dough with egg wash. Bake the pie at 350° F/177° C for 55 to 60 minutes, until the filling begins to bubble slightly.

Cane-Sugar-Free Fruit Pie:

Make this pie early on the day it is to be served for a firm filling. Sprinkle ¼ cup (30 g) of tapioca starch on 5 cups (700 g) of fruit of choice (berries, peeled and sliced apples, etc.); if using apples, also sprinkle with 1 t. (3 g) cinnamon. Gently mix till all of the fruit is coated with the starch. In a small bowl, mix together ½ cup (125 g) unsweetened applesauce and 45 drops of clear, alcohol-free liquid stevia; add this mixture to the fruit and mix gently. Follow either the Double-crust Pie Dough or Faux Double-crust Pie recipe above for preparing the pie crust. Bake in a 350° F/177° C oven for 45 to 60 minutes, till the filling begins to bubble slightly. Cool to room temperature before serving.

Cookies and Treats

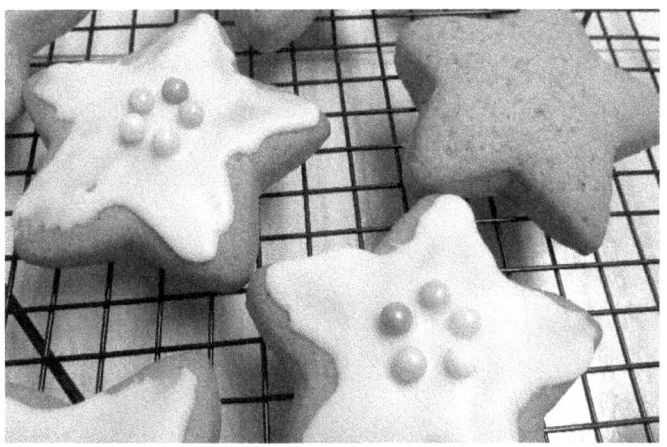

Chocolate Chip Cookies

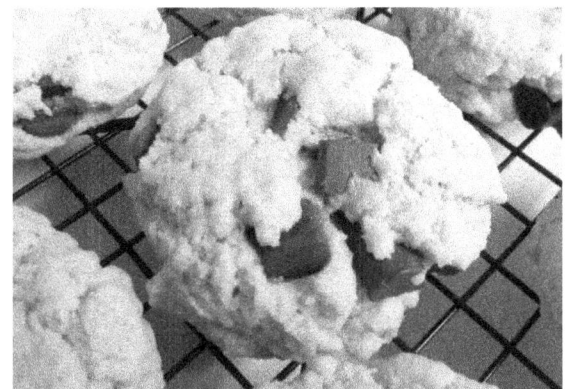

These cookies can be made as either bar cookies or drop cookies. For a richer and chewier cookie, add 1 Tablespoon (15 ml) of rice syrup or corn syrup in Step 2. Makes about 2 dozen drop cookies or 9 bar cookies.

☑ Allergy/Intolerance Substitutions:
Eggs: Prepare the equivalent of one egg using the Non-rising Egg Replacer (page 76) or Chia Seed Egg Replacer (page 74). In step 2, leave out the egg and add the egg replacer.

☑ Reduced Sugar:
In step 1, leave out the sugar. In step 2, add to the liquid ingredients 70 drops of clear, alcohol-free liquid stevia, 1 T. (15 ml) almond extract (if tolerated), and an extra 2 T. (30 ml) milk of choice (i.e., ¼ cup or 59 ml milk of choice total). In step 3, use sugar-free GF-DF-SF chocolate or carob chips.

Dough Ingredients:
1½ c. gluten-free flour mix (195 g)
½ c. refined cane sugar (100 g)
⅛ t. salt (0.7 g)
1 large egg
1 T. vanilla extract (15 ml)
2 T. milk of choice (30 ml)
½ c. shortening or lard, melted (72 g)
½ c. GF-DF-SF chocolate chips (90 g)

Preheat Oven: 350° F/177° C

Directions:
Step 1. Mix together the gluten-free flour mix, sugar, and salt.

Step 2. In a small mixing bowl, whisk together the egg, vanilla, milk of choice, and melted shortening/lard. Add this mixture to the dry ingredients, mixing well with a rubber spatula until a stiff dough forms and all of the flour is incorporated into the dough.

Step 3. Mix in the chocolate chips. Let the dough rest at room temperature for five minutes.

Step 4. *For bar cookies:* Spray a square 8" x 8" (20 cm x 20 cm) pan with cooking oil. Press the cookie dough evenly into the pan. Bake 18 to 22 minutes, till the cookies are golden brown. Remove the pan from the oven and cool for 10 minutes; slice into bars.

For drop cookies: Line two cookie sheets with parchment paper. For each cookie, scoop the dough with a small cookie dough scoop, and then roll the dough between your hands to form a ball. Place the dough balls on a cookie sheet, spacing them about two inches apart and flattening them slightly with your fingertips. Bake the cookies for 12 to 15 minutes till golden brown on the bottom. Remove the pans from the oven and cool for 3 minutes. Use a metal spatula to move the cookies to a cooling rack.

Nutritional content (bar cookies): Makes 9 servings (1 bar (67 g) per serving). Each serving contains: Calories (280); Total Fat (14 g); Saturated Fat (6 g); Cholesterol (20 mg); Sodium (160 mg); Potassium (83 mg); Total Carbohydrate (38 g); Dietary Fiber (1 g); Sugars (17 g); Protein (2 g). Nutrient(s) of note (percent of Daily Value): Calcium 2%, Iron 4%

Nutritional content (drop cookies): Makes 24 servings (1 cookie (25 g) per serving). Each serving contains: Calories (100); Total Fat (5 g); Saturated Fat (2.5 g); Cholesterol (10 mg); Sodium (60 mg); Potassium (31 mg); Total Carbohydrate (14 g); Dietary Fiber (0 g); Sugars (6 g); Protein (1 g). Nutrient(s) of note (percent of Daily Value): Iron 2%

Chocolate Chip Cookie Cups:

Follow the Chocolate Chip Cookie recipe through Step 3. Spray the cups of a mini muffin pan with cooking spray. Press 1 Tablespoon (17 g) of dough into each cup of the mini muffin pan, forming a cup shape with the dough. Bake at 415° F/213° C for about 12 minutes. Remove from the oven. If the cookie cups have puffed up during baking, gently reopen the cups with the tip of a knife to reform the cup shape. Cool to room temperature in the muffin pan, and then place the muffin pan in the freezer for 1 hour. Remove the pan from the freezer. Using a pastry decorating bag, fill the cookie cups with Chocolate Coconut Ganache (see page 249). Place in a cool location (not the refrigerator) overnight to solidify the ganache. Gently remove the cookie cups from the pan and enjoy!

Not-So-Plain Sugar Cookies

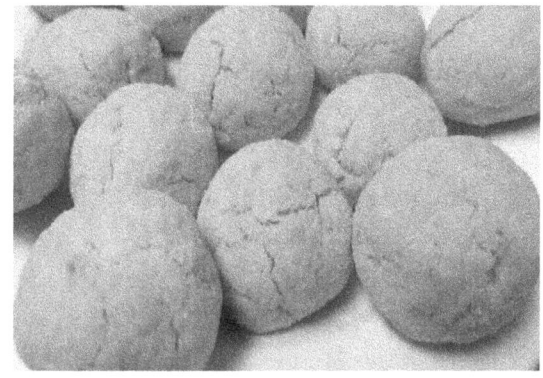

Though simple in appearance, these cookies are delicious — light in texture, with a thin, crisp crust of sugar on the outside and a mild orange flavor. This recipe uses almond meal to keep the cookies moist. Excellent warm out of the oven! For a special touch, insert a chocolate chunk inside each dough ball prior to baking (make sure the chocolate is completely encased in the dough). Makes about 2 dozen.

☑ **Allergy/Intolerance Substitutions:**
Tree nuts: In step 1, replace the almond meal with pumpkin seed meal or sunflower seed meal. In step 2, replace the almond extract with an equal measure of vanilla extract.
Eggs: Prepare the equivalent of one egg using the Non-rising Egg Replacer (page 76). In step 2, leave out the egg and add the egg replacer.

☑ **Reduced Sugar:**
In step 1, leave out the sugar. In step 2, add 75 to 80 drops of clear, alcohol-free liquid stevia, and one extra egg or egg replacer (i.e., two eggs or egg replacers total). Knead the dough till it pulls together. In step 5, roll the dough

balls in finely chopped nuts (if tolerated) instead of the 3 T. (37 g) sugar. Bake as directed.

Dough Ingredients:
1½ c. gluten-free flour mix (195 g)
½ c. almond meal (50 g)
1 t. baking powder (5 g)
½ c. plus 3 T. refined cane sugar (100 g plus 37 g)
⅛ t. salt (0.7 g)
1 large egg
1 T. almond extract (15 ml)
1 T. orange extract (15 ml)
1 T. fresh orange zest (6 g)
½ c. shortening or lard (72 g), melted

Preheat Oven: 350° F/177° C

Directions:
Step 1. In a large mixing bowl, combine the gluten-free flour mix, almond meal, baking powder, ½ cup (100 g) of sugar, and salt.

Step 2. In a small mixing bowl, whisk together the egg, almond extract, orange extract and zest, and melted shortening/lard. Add this mixture to the dry ingredients and combine with a rubber spatula to form a stiff dough. Shape the dough into a ball, wrap it in wax paper, and place it in the refrigerator for 20 minutes.

Step 3. Place the remaining 3 T. (37 g) of sugar in a shallow dish or bowl.

Step 4. Line a cookie sheet with parchment paper. Spray the paper with cooking spray.

Step 5. Scoop out some dough with a small cookie dough scoop, leveling off the dough with a knife or on the edge of the mixing bowl. Remove the dough from the cookie scoop and roll it in your hands to form a ball. Roll the ball in the dish of sugar, and place it on the parchment-lined cookie sheet. Repeat till all of the dough is used, spacing the balls about one inch (2.5 cm) apart on the cookie sheet.

Step 6. Place the cookie sheet in the oven, and bake for about 15 minutes till the cookies are slightly golden brown on the bottom.

Step 7. Remove the cookie sheet from the oven. Use a metal spatula to move the cookies to a cooling rack. Enjoy these cookies either warm or at room temperature.

Nutritional content: Makes 24 servings (1 cookie (25 g) per serving). Each serving contains: Calories (110); Total Fat (6 g); Saturated Fat (2 g); Cholesterol (10 mg); Sodium (85 mg); Potassium (10 mg); Total Carbohydrate (13 g); Dietary Fiber (1 g); Sugars (5 g); Protein (1 g). Nutrient(s) of note (percent of Daily Value): Calcium 2%, Iron 2%

Honey & Spice Cookies

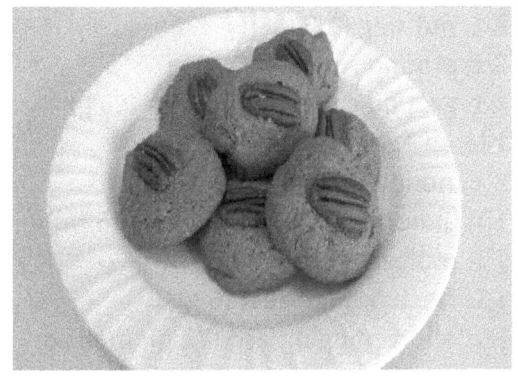

These cane-sugar-free cookies taste like gingerbread, and have a light, cake-like texture. The touch of cayenne pepper gives them a little kick. Drizzle with Orange-flavored Icing (see page 255) for an extra burst of flavor. Makes about 2 dozen.

☑ **Allergy/Intolerance Substitutions:**
Tree nuts: Use vanilla extract instead of almond extract in step 2. Leave out the whole pecans in step 5.
Eggs: Prepare the equivalent of one egg using the Non-rising Egg Replacer (page 76). In step 2, leave out the egg and add the egg replacer.
Nightshade family: In step 1, leave out the cayenne pepper.

☑ **Reduced Sugar:**
In step 2, leave out the honey and molasses. Add 70 to 80 drops of clear, alcohol-free liquid stevia and 6 T. (90 ml) milk of choice. If using egg replacer, you may need to add an extra 1 to 2 T. (15 to 30 ml) milk of choice to make the dough pliable. These cookies will not brown due to the absence of the honey; be careful not to overbake.

Dough Ingredients:
1½ c. gluten-free flour mix (195 g)
½ t. baking powder (2.5 g)
⅛ t. salt (0.7 g)
2 t. ground dried ginger (6 g)
1 t. cinnamon (3 g)
½ t. nutmeg (1.5 g)
¼ t. ground cloves (0.7 g)
⅛ t. ground cayenne pepper (0.3 g)
1 large egg
½ c. honey (174 g)
1 T. almond or vanilla extract (15 ml)
1 T. molasses (15 ml)
1 T. fresh orange zest (6 g)
½ c. shortening or lard (72 g), melted
½ c. whole pecans (optional) (45 g)

Preheat Oven: 350° F/177° C

Directions:
Step 1. In a large bowl, mix together the gluten-free flour mix, baking powder, salt, ginger, cinnamon, nutmeg, ground cloves, and cayenne pepper.

Step 2. In a small mixing bowl, whisk together the egg, honey, almond or vanilla extract, molasses, orange zest, and melted shortening/lard. Add this mixture to the dry ingredients, mixing with a rubber spatula till a smooth, sticky dough forms. Let the dough rest, uncovered, at room temperature for 15 minutes.

Step 3. Line two cookie sheets with parchment paper and spray with cooking oil.

Step 4. Scoop out some dough with a small cookie dough scoop, scraping the excess dough off with a knife or on the edge of the mixing bowl. Place the ball of dough on a cookie sheet. Gently smooth the top and sides of the cookie with your fingertips. Repeat for the other cookies, spacing them about two inches apart on the cookie sheets.

Step 5. Press a whole pecan firmly into the top of each cookie (optional).

Step 6. Place the cookie sheets in the oven and bake about 12 minutes till the cookies are golden brown. Remove the cookie sheets from the oven and let cool for one minute. Use a metal spatula to move the cookies to a cooling rack. For an extra burst of flavor, drizzle with Orange-flavored Icing (see page 255) after they have completely cooled.

Nutritional content: Makes 24 servings (1 cookie (26 g) per serving; includes pecans but excludes icing). Each serving contains: Calories (110); Total Fat (6 g); Saturated Fat (2 g); Cholesterol (10 mg); Sodium (75 mg); Potassium (35 mg); Total Carbohydrate (14 g); Dietary Fiber (1 g); Sugars (6 g); Protein (1 g). Nutrient(s) of note (percent of Daily Value): Iron 2%

Gingerbread Cookies

Though similar in taste to the Honey and Spice Cookies, these cookies contain bean flour which makes it possible to roll out the dough and shape it with a cookie cutter. Because the dough is rolled out between two pieces of plastic wrap rather than on a floured surface, the dough scraps can be kneaded back together and rolled out repeatedly till all of the dough has been used. These cookies are delicious frosted with Orange-flavored Icing (see photo; page 255).

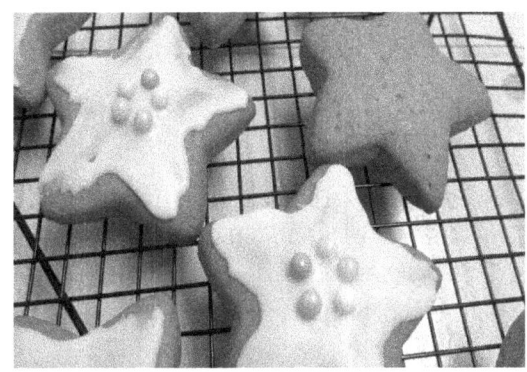

☑ Allergy/Intolerance Substitutions:
Tree nuts: In step 2, use vanilla extract instead of almond extract.

Eggs: Prepare the equivalent of one egg using the Non-rising Egg Replacer (page 76). In step 2, leave out the egg and add the egg replacer.

☑ Reduced Sugar:
In step 2, leave out the honey and molasses; add 80 drops of clear, alcohol-free liquid stevia and 6 T. (90 ml) milk of choice. If the dough cracks easily when rolled out, add an extra 1 to 2 T. (15 to 30 ml) milk of choice. These cookies will not brown due to the absence of the honey; do not over bake.

Dough Ingredients:
1½ c. gluten-free flour mix (195 g)
½ c. fava or garbanzo bean flour (52 g)
⅛ t. salt (0.7 g)
2 t. ground dried ginger (6 g)
1 t. cinnamon (3 g)
½ t. nutmeg (1.5 g)
¼ t. ground cloves (0.7 g)
⅛ t. ground cayenne pepper (0.3 g)
1 large egg
½ c. honey (174 g)
1 T. almond or vanilla extract (15 ml)
1 T. molasses (15 ml)
1 T. fresh orange zest (6 g)
½ c. shortening or lard, melted (72 g)

Preheat Oven: 350° F/177° C

Directions:
Step 1. In a large bowl, mix together the gluten-free flour mix, bean flour, salt, ginger, cinnamon, nutmeg, ground cloves, and cayenne pepper.

Step 2. In a small mixing bowl, whisk together the egg, honey, almond or vanilla extract, molasses, orange zest, and melted shortening/lard. Add this mixture to the dry ingredients, mixing well with a rubber spatula to form a sticky dough. Shape the dough into a ball and wrap it in wax paper. Place the dough ball in the refrigerator for 30 minutes.

Step 3. Line two cookie sheets with parchment paper.

Step 4. Remove the dough ball from the refrigerator, unwrap it, and divide it in half. Roll out half of the dough between two sheets of plastic wrap with a rolling pin till the dough is ¼-inch (0.6-cm) thick. Remove the top sheet of plastic wrap and cut the dough with a cookie cutter. Carefully lift the cookie cutter (with the dough attached) off the bottom layer of plastic wrap. Gently push the cookie dough out of the cookie cutter onto a parchment-lined cookie sheet. If the dough sticks to the bottom layer of plastic wrap, gently peel the dough off the plastic wrap and place it on the cookie sheet. Use the cookie cutter on the rest of the dough, leaving a one-inch (2.5 cm) space between the cookies on the cookie sheets. Repeat this step for the other half of the dough.

Step 5. Knead together the scraps of leftover dough. Roll-out between two sheets of plastic wrap and cut out more cookies. Repeat this step till all of the dough has been used.

Step 6. Bake for 9 to 11 minutes. Remove the cookie sheets from the oven and cool for one minute. Use a metal spatula to move the cookies to a cooling rack. When completely cool, frost and decorate with GF-DF-SF sprinkles.

Nutritional content: Makes 15 servings (1 cookie (32 g) per serving; excludes icing). Each serving contains: Calories (140); Total Fat (8 g); Saturated Fat (3.5 g); Cholesterol (10 mg); Sodium (100 mg); Potassium (46 mg); Total Carbohydrate (16 g); Dietary Fiber (2 g); Sugars (1 g); Protein (2 g). Nutrient(s) of note (percent of Daily Value): Calcium 2%, Vitamin C 2%, Iron 4%

All-But-The-Kitchen-Sink Bars

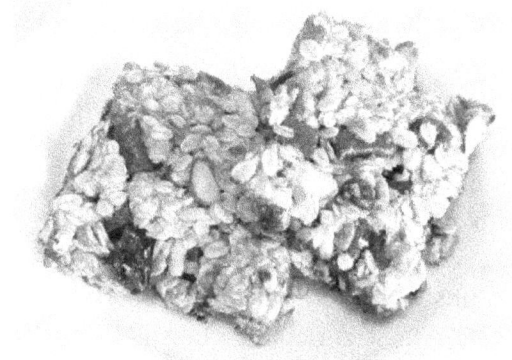

Packed with oats, nuts, chocolate chips, and dried fruit, these chewy bars are great for picnics and day hikes, or for boxed lunches. If you want to make them less chewy, leave out the corn syrup or rice syrup. Makes about 15 bars.

☑ **Allergy/Intolerance Substitutions:**
Corn: In step 2, use an additive-free rice syrup in place of the corn syrup.
Coconut: In step 4, leave out the shredded coconut (no replacement necessary).
Tree nuts: In step 4, leave out the sliced almonds (no replacement needed), or replace with ¼ cup (25 g) pumpkin seeds.
Eggs: Prepare the equivalent of two whole eggs using the Flax Meal, Chia Seed, or Non-rising Egg Replacer (pages 73-76). In step 2, leave out the egg whites and add the egg replacer.
Oats: Avoid this recipe.
Rice: In step 2, use corn syrup in place of rice syrup.

☑ **Reduced Sugar:**
No suggestions given; this recipe does not come out well without the brown sugar, and rice or corn syrup.

Dough Ingredients:
½ c. gluten-free flour mix (65 g)
½ c. lightly-packed brown sugar (72 g)
¼ t. salt (1.5 g)
¼ c. brown rice syrup or light corn syrup (59 ml)
¼ c. pure olive oil (not extra virgin) or other neutral-flavored oil (59 ml)
2 egg whites
2½ c. certified GF rolled oats (250 g)
¼ c. unsweetened shredded coconut (18 g)
½ c. GF-DF-SF chocolate chips (90 g)
¼ c. dried cranberries (40 g)
¼ c. sliced almonds (25 g)
¼ c. sunflower seeds (25 g)

Preheat Oven: 325° F/163° C

Directions:
Step 1. In a large mixing bowl, combine the gluten-free flour mix, brown sugar, and salt.

Step 2. Add the rice or corn syrup, oil, and egg whites to the dry ingredients. Mix with a rubber spatula to form a smooth paste.

Step 3. Add in the oats, combining thoroughly with the rubber spatula to coat all of the oats with the sugar, flour, and syrup mixture.

Step 4. Mix in the remaining ingredients.

Step 5. Line a 9" x 13" (23 cm x 33 cm) pan with parchment paper; the paper should extend at least one inch above the pan on two opposite sides (see photo insert). Spray the paper in the bottom of the pan with cooking spray.

Spread the mixture evenly in the paper-lined pan. Push down on the dough with a rubber spatula to compact it; the mixture should be about ½ inch (1 cm) thick when done.

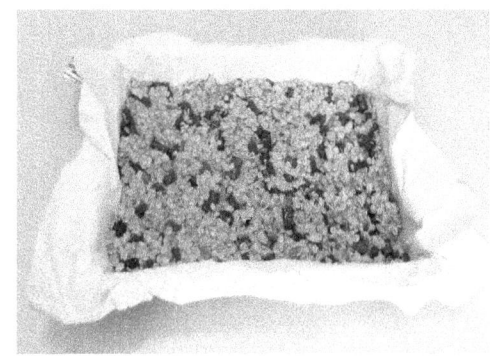

Step 6. Bake for about 27 to 30 minutes until the top of the bars turn golden brown and no longer look raw.

Step 7. Remove the pan from the oven. Gently remove the bars from the pan by lifting the opposite sides of the parchment paper; place the bars (with the parchment paper beneath) flat on a cutting board. Cool for 20 minutes.

Step 8. Use a serrated knife to cut into bars. Let the bars cool completely on the cutting board before moving them to a container for storage.

Nutritional content: Makes 15 servings (1 bar (56 g) per serving). Each serving contains: Calories (220); Total Fat (9 g); Saturated Fat (2.5 g); Cholesterol (0 mg); Sodium (85 mg); Potassium (91 mg); Total Carbohydrate (31 g); Dietary Fiber (3 g); Sugars (13 g); Protein (5 g). Nutrient(s) of note (percent of Daily Value): Calcium 2%, Iron 8%

Old-fashioned Oatmeal Cookies

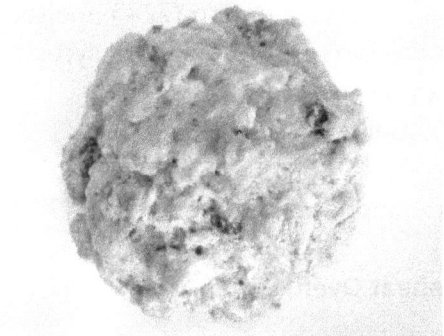

These cookies are chewy and crisp, with a light cinnamon flavor. If you prefer a sweeter cookie, replace the raisins with GF-DF-SF chocolate chips or GF-SF butterscotch chips (for those who tolerate dairy only). Makes about 15 large cookies.

☑ **Allergy/Intolerance Substitutions:**
Corn: In step 3, use an additive-free brown rice syrup instead of corn syrup.
Tree nuts: In step 4, leave out the pecans (no replacement needed).
Eggs: Prepare the equivalent of two eggs using the Non-rising Egg Replacer (page 76). In step 3, leave out the eggs and add 5 T. (75 ml) of the egg replacer.
Oats: Avoid this recipe.
Rice: In step 3, use corn syrup instead of rice syrup.

☑ **Reduced Sugar:**
No suggestions given; this recipe does not work well without the brown sugar, and rice or corn syrup.

Dough Ingredients:
1 c. gluten-free flour mix (130 g)
½ c. lightly-packed brown sugar (72 g)
½ t. cinnamon (1.5 g)
⅛ t. salt (0.7 g)
1½ c. certified GF rolled oats (150 g)
½ c. shortening or lard (72 g), melted
¼ c. brown rice syrup or corn syrup (59 ml)
2 large eggs
1 T. vanilla extract (15 ml)
½ c. raisins (80 g)
¼ c. chopped pecans (optional) (25 g)

Preheat Oven: 350° F/177° C

Directions:
Step 1. In a large mixing bowl, combine the gluten-free flour mix, brown sugar, cinnamon, and salt with a rubber spatula, breaking up any clumps of brown sugar.

Step 2. Mix in the oats.

Step 3. Add the melted shortening/lard, rice or corn syrup, eggs, and vanilla extract. Thoroughly combine with a rubber spatula till a thick, sticky dough forms and all of the flour is completely incorporated into the dough.

Step 4. Mix in the raisins and pecans. Let the dough rest at room temperature for 15 minutes.

Step 5. Line two cookie sheets with parchment paper. Spray the paper with cooking spray.

Step 6. Scoop out some dough with a large cookie dough scoop, scraping off the excess dough with a knife or on the edge of the mixing bowl. (Note: you may need to push the dough into the scoop with your fingertips to get a full scoop.) Release the dough from the scoop directly onto the parchment (because the dough is sticky, you may need to gently pull the dough out of the scoop). Repeat this step for the other cookies, spacing them about two inches apart on the cookie sheets. Gently flatten the cookies with your fingertips till each is about ½-inch (1 cm) thick.

Step 7. Place the cookie sheets in the oven. Bake for 15 to 18 minutes till the cookies are golden brown. Remove from the oven and cool for one minute. Use a metal spatula to move the cookies to a cooling rack. Enjoy either warm or at room temperature.

Nutritional content: Makes 15 servings (1 cookie (54 g) per serving; includes raisins and pecans). Each serving contains: Calories (220); Total Fat (10 g); Saturated Fat (3.5 g); Cholesterol (25 mg); Sodium (90 mg); Potassium (85 mg); Total Carbohydrate (31 g); Dietary Fiber (2 g); Sugars (13 g); Protein (3 g). Nutrient(s) of note (percent of Daily Value): Calcium 2%, Iron 6%

Super Rich Brownies

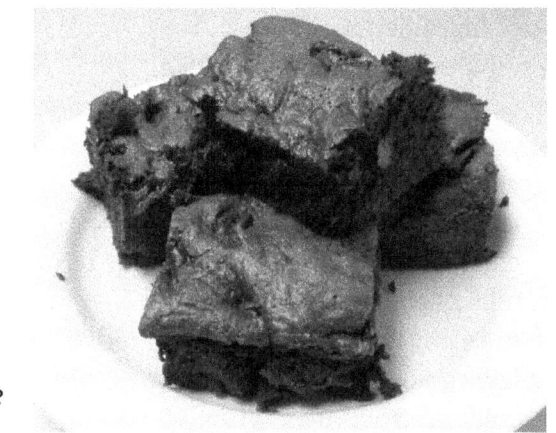

These brownies are very chocolaty and have a rich, cake-like consistency. For a brownie sundae, serve warm with some Frozen Coconut Vanilla Custard and drizzle with warm Chocolate Coconut Ganache (see the last chapter for these recipes). For chewier and flatter brownies, leave out one of the eggs.

☑ Allergy/Intolerance Substitutions:
Corn: In step 2, use an additive-free brown rice syrup in place of the corn syrup.
Eggs: Prepare the equivalent of two eggs using the Rising Egg Replacer for cakes (page 74). In step 2, leave out the eggs and add the egg replacer (be sure to add the apple cider vinegar as specified in the egg replacer recipe).
Rice: In step 2, use corn syrup in place of the rice syrup.

☑ Reduced Sugar:
In step 1, add to the dry ingredients ¼ cup (26 g) bean flour or quinoa flour, and ¼ cup (25 g) almond meal, pumpkin seed meal, or sunflower seed meal. In step 2, leave out the sugar or honey, as well as the corn syrup or

rice syrup. Add 85 drops of clear, alcohol-free liquid stevia and ½ cup (125 g) unsweetened applesauce. Replace the 1 t. (5 ml) vanilla extract with 1 T. (15 ml) vanilla extract. In step 3, use sugar-free GF-DF-SF chocolate or carob chips, or leave out completely.

Batter Ingredients:
1½ c. gluten-free flour mix (195 g)
½ c. GF-DF-SF unsweetened cocoa powder (50 g)
¼ t. salt (1.5 g)
2 large eggs
½ c. refined cane sugar (100 g) or honey (174 g)
½ c. corn syrup or brown rice syrup (118 ml)
¼ c. milk of choice (59 ml)
¾ c. pure olive oil (not extra virgin) or other neutral-flavored oil (177 ml)
1 t. vanilla extract (5 ml)
½ c. GF-DF-SF chocolate chips (optional) (90 g)

Preheat Oven: 375° F/191° C

Directions:
Step 1. In a large mixing bowl, combine the gluten-free flour mix, cocoa, and salt.

Step 2. In a small mixing bowl, whisk together the eggs, sugar or honey, corn syrup or rice syrup, milk of choice, oil, and vanilla extract. Add this mixture to the dry ingredients; stir with a rubber spatula to form a smooth, thick batter.

Step 3. Stir in the chocolate chips.

Step 4. For thinner brownies, spray cooking oil in a 9" x 13" (23 cm x 33 cm) baking pan; for thicker brownies, spray an 8" x 8" (20 cm x 20 cm) pan. Pour the batter into the pan and spread it evenly with a rubber spatula.

Step 5. Bake for 20 to 25 minutes for the 9" x 13" (23 cm x 33 cm) baking pan, or 25 to 30 minutes for the 8" x 8" (20 cm x 20 cm) pan. Cool and cut into squares.

Nutritional content: Makes 15 servings (1 brownie (64 g) per serving, using a 9" x 13" pan (23 cm x 33 cm)). Each serving contains: Calories (250); Total Fat (13 g); Saturated Fat (2.5 g); Cholesterol (25 mg); Sodium (105 mg); Potassium (126 mg); Total Carbohydrate (34 g); Dietary Fiber (2 g); Sugars (16 g); Protein (2 g). Nutrient(s) of note (percent of Daily Value): Calcium 2%, Iron 6%

Basil's Chocolate Biscotti

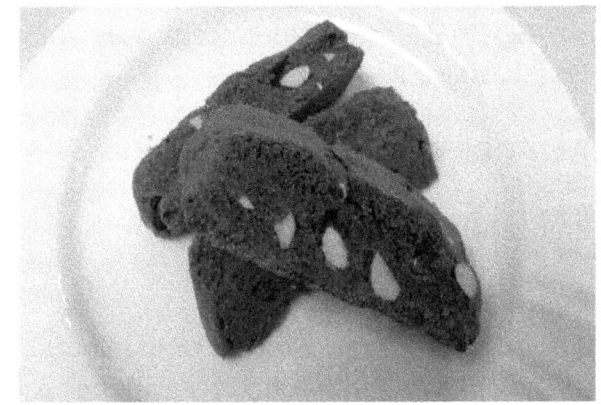

Biscotti are dry Italian cookies perfect for dipping into coffee or hot cocoa. Being of Italian heritage, the day that I figured out I could make biscotti that taste the same as the original was a very good day. The original biscotti recipe came from a dear friend of my family's, Basil Fabbioli; my adapted version is below.

☑ Allergy/Intolerance Substitutions:
Tree nuts: In steps 1 and 5, leave out the nuts (no replacement needed), or add shelled sunflower seeds instead (if tolerated).
Eggs: Prepare the equivalent of 2 eggs using the Non-rising Egg Replacer (page 76). In step 2, leave out the eggs and add the egg replacer.

☑ Reduced Sugar:
No suggestions given; this recipe does not work well without the sugar.

Dough Ingredients:
½ c. whole raw almonds or hazelnuts (optional) (80 g)
½ c. shortening or lard (72 g)
¾ c. refined cane sugar (150 g)
2 large eggs
2¼ c. gluten-free flour mix (292 g)
⅓ c. GF-DF-SF unsweetened cocoa powder (34 g)
1½ t. baking powder (7.5 g)
¼ t. salt (1.5 g)
½ c. GF-DF-SF chocolate chips (90 g)

Preheat Oven: 325° F/163° C

Directions:
Step 1. Roast the raw almonds or hazelnuts in a baking pan for 10 minutes. Let the nuts cool and then chop them into large pieces.

Step 2. In a large mixing bowl, cream together the lard/shortening, sugar, and eggs with an electric mixer.

Step 3. In another bowl, mix together the gluten-free flour mix, cocoa powder, baking powder, and salt.

Step 4. Gradually add the dry ingredients to the creamed mixture, mixing well with an electric mixer till a thick and crumbly dough forms (the dough will pull together as you knead it in step 5). Scrape the sides of the bowl with a rubber spatula and mix for another 30 seconds.

Step 5. Add in the nuts and chocolate chips. Knead the dough with your hands to form a smooth, chunky dough.

Step 6. Line a cookie sheet with non-stick aluminum foil (non-stick side facing up). Divide the dough into four, equally-sized pieces. Roll each piece between your hands into a log that is about 2 inches (5 cm) in diameter. Place the log onto the aluminum foil-covered cookie sheet and gently flatten it into a rectangle that is roughly ¾-inch (2 cm) thick, 3 inches (7.5 cm) wide, and about 6 inches (15 cm) long. Repeat this process for the other three pieces of dough, spacing them at least 2 inches (5 cm) apart on the cookie sheet.

Step 7. Bake for 25 minutes.

Step 8. Remove the pan from the oven. Gently remove the logs from the cookie sheet with a metal spatula, and place them on a cooling rack. Cool for 5 minutes.

Step 9. Move one log to a cutting board. With a heavy, sharp, serrated knife, carefully slice the log (holding the knife at a 45-degree angle and perpendicular to the length of the log) into ¾-inch (2 cm) thick slices. The nuts make these slices difficult to cut without breaking. The trick is to cut halfway down through the log using a gentle sawing motion, and then use the weight of the knife to push down through the rest of the log. Lay the slices of biscotti flat on the cookie sheet. Repeat this process for the other logs.

Step 10. Bake the biscotti slices for 10 to 12 minutes till the middle of the biscotti appear slightly dry.

Step 11. Remove the cookie sheet from the oven. Using a metal spatula, move the biscotti to a cooling rack. When completely cool, the biscotti can be stored in a tightly sealed container at room temperature for one week.

Nutritional content: Makes 24 servings (1 cookie (37 g) per serving). Each serving contains: Calories (150); Total Fat (7 g); Saturated Fat (2.5 g); Cholesterol (15 mg); Sodium (135 mg); Potassium (75 mg); Total Carbohydrate (21 g); Dietary Fiber (1 g); Sugars (8 g); Protein (2 g). Nutrient(s) of note (percent of Daily Value): Calcium 2%, Iron 4%

Try a Different Flavor of Biscotti:

In step 2, add 1½ Tablespoons (22 ml) of anise, almond, or vanilla extract. In step 3, leave out the cocoa powder and reduce the amount of baking powder to 1 teaspoon (5 g). In step 5, leave out the chocolate chips if needed. Follow the directions for baking in steps 6 to 11.

"Butter" Cookies

These cookies taste buttery due to the addition of imitation, non-dairy butter flavor (available in most grocery stores in the baking aisle). If you wish to avoid using the non-dairy butter flavor, simply replace it with 1 t. (5 ml) pure maple syrup

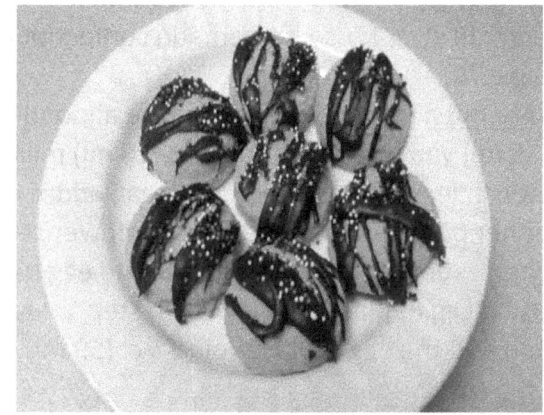

plus 1 t. (5 ml) vanilla extract. These cookies have a slightly salty aftertaste which pairs well with sweet chocolate frostings; if you wish to eat the cookies plain or with a vanilla frosting, use only ½ t. (3 g) salt in step 2 instead of the full teaspoon (6 g) listed in the recipe below.

To decorate these cookies for holidays or parties, mix Vanilla Icing (see page 255) with GF-DF-SF food color, ice the cookies, and immediately top with GF-DF-SF sprinkles, chopped nuts, or mini GF-DF-SF chocolate chips. This recipe can also be used to make great "half-moon" cookies; simply use a large cookie dough scoop to prepare the dough balls in step 3, and decorate the cooled cookies with half chocolate and half vanilla frosting (see the last chapter for these recipes). You can also sprinkle on a coarse sugar prior to baking, or drizzle the baked and cooled cookies with Chocolate Coconut Ganache (see photo insert and recipe on page 249). Prior to frosting, these cookies can be frozen for up to a month (be sure to wrap them well in wax paper to prevent freezer burn). Make sure that the sprinkles or other decorations you use are free of any allergens of concern.

☑ Allergy/Intolerance Substitutions:

<u>Corn:</u> In step 1, use homemade confectioner's sugar (see page 70).

<u>Tree nuts:</u> In step 1, leave out the almond extract; add 1 T. (15 ml) vanilla extract and 1 T. (15 ml) milk of choice. In step 2, leave out the almond meal; add ¼ cup (25 g) of either pumpkin seed meal or sunflower seed meal.

<u>Eggs:</u> Prepare the equivalent of one egg using the Non-rising Egg Replacer (page 76). In step 1, leave out the egg, and add the egg replacer plus ¼ c. (59 ml) milk of choice.

☑ Reduced Sugar:

None; this recipe does not turn out well without the confectioner's sugar.

Dough Ingredients:

1 c. shortening or lard (144 g)
1 c. confectioner's sugar (120 g)
1 large egg
1 T. almond extract (15 ml)
1 t. GF-DF-SF imitation butter flavoring (5 ml)
2½ c. gluten-free flour mix (325 g)
¼ c. almond meal (25 g)
1 t. salt (6 g) (reduce to ½ t. (3 g) for plain or vanilla-frosted cookies)

Preheat Oven: 325° F/163° C

Directions:

Step 1. In a large mixing bowl, cream together the shortening/lard, confectioner's sugar, egg, almond extract, and imitation butter flavor with an electric mixer.

Step 2. In a medium-sized bowl, mix together the gluten-free flour mix, almond meal, and salt. Add this flour mixture gradually to the shortening/egg mixture, beating with the electric mixer after each addition. Scrape the sides of the mixing bowl with a rubber spatula, and then beat the mixture for another minute. The mixture will be crumbly at this point; knead it for one minute to pull it together into a ball shape. If the dough does not easily come together into a ball, add 1 T. (15 ml) milk of choice, beat for another minute, and then form it into a ball. Let the dough rest at room temperature for five minutes.

Step 3. Line two cookie sheets with parchment paper. Scoop out some dough with a small cookie dough scoop, leveling the dough off by scraping it with a knife or on the edge of the mixing bowl. Release the ball of dough from the scoop, roll it gently in your hands to smooth, and place it on a cookie sheet. Repeat for the other cookies. Space the cookies about 2 inches (5 cm) apart on the cookie sheets.

Step 4. Bake for 14 to 15 minutes, till the bottom edges of the cookies turn a light golden brown. Do not over-bake! Using a metal spatula, move the cookies from the cookie sheets to a wire rack to cool.

Step 5. After the cookies have cooled, decorate with icing, GF-DF-SF sprinkles, chopped nuts, or chocolate chips (optional). Place the cookies in a dark, cool location (not the refrigerator) overnight to harden the frosting or ganache.

Nutritional content: Makes 24 servings (1 small cookie (33 g) per serving; excludes frosting and decorations). Each serving contains: Calories (160); Total Fat (10 g); Saturated Fat (4 g); Cholesterol (10 mg); Sodium (230 mg); Potassium (14 mg); Total Carbohydrate (18 g); Dietary Fiber (1 g); Sugars (5 g); Protein (1 g). Nutrient(s) of note (percent of Daily Value): Iron 2%

Fried Dough

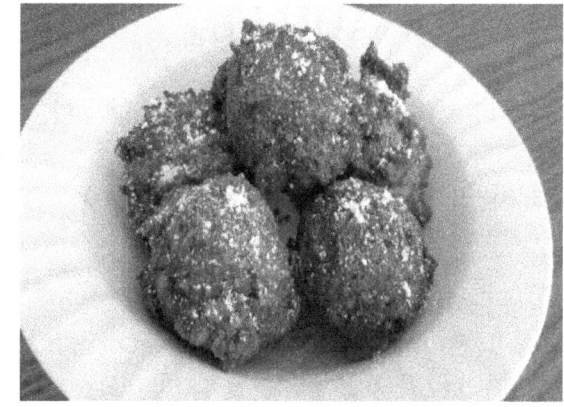

*E*very time I go to our State Fair and feel deprived over not being able to eat the fried dough, I make these. These are so tasty that it's hard to eat just one. They taste best warm. The reduced sugar recipe comes out as well as the original, though slightly less sweet. Make sure that rapid rise yeast is used, since active dry yeast does not work well with this recipe. The oils that work best for deep frying the dough balls are pure olive (not extra virgin), safflower, or sunflower. Makes about 1 dozen.

☑ **Allergy/Intolerance Substitutions:**
Corn: In step 9, sprinkle with homemade confectioner's sugar made with tapioca starch (see page 70).
Eggs: Prepare the equivalent of one egg using the Non-rising Egg Replacer (page 76). In step 3, leave out the egg and add the egg replacer.
Yeast: Avoid this recipe.

☑ **Reduced Sugar:**
In step 2, leave out the sugar and add an extra ½ t. (1.5 g) cinnamon (i.e., ¾ t. or 4.5 g cinnamon total). In step 3, add

¼ cup (62 g) unsweetened applesauce and 20 to 25 drops of clear, alcohol-free liquid stevia.

Dough Ingredients:
2 quarts oil for deep frying (1.9 liters)
1½ c. gluten-free flour mix (195 g)
½ c. refined cane sugar (100 g)
¼ t. cinnamon (0.7 g)
2¼ t. (one packet) rapid rise yeast (8.5 g)
1 large egg
1 T. vanilla extract (15 ml)
½ c. hot tap water (118 ml)

Directions:
Step 1. Pour the oil into a large sauce pan until it's about one inch (2.5 cm) deep. Heat the oil over medium heat till it reaches a temperature of 350° F/177° C.

Step 2. As the oil is heating, mix together the gluten-free flour mix, sugar, cinnamon, and yeast in a medium-sized bowl.

Step 3. In a small mixing bowl, whisk together the egg, vanilla extract, and hot tap water.

Step 4. Add the egg/water mixture to the dry ingredients. Mix with an electric mixer till a smooth, thick, and sticky dough forms. Scrape the sides and bottom of the bowl, and mix for another 30 seconds.

Step 5. Let the dough rest, uncovered, for ten minutes to activate the yeast.

Step 6. You will need to fry these donuts in two separate batches. Scoop up 1 T. (17 g) of dough (about the size of a golf ball) with a spoon; scrape the dough off the spoon and into the heated oil using a rubber spatula. Repeat for four to five other dough balls, reserving about half of the dough for a second batch. Using a slotted metal spoon, gently separate the dough balls in the hot oil to prevent them from sticking together.

Step 7. Cook the dough balls in the hot oil for 1½ to 2 minutes till the bottom of each ball turns a deep golden brown. Using the slotted spoon, gently flip the dough balls and cook the other side for another 1½ to 2 minutes till deep golden brown. Carefully remove the balls from the hot oil with the slotted spoon and place them on a paper-lined plate to drain.

Step 8. Bring the temperature of the oil back to 350° F/ 177° C. Repeat steps 6 and 7 for the second batch of fried dough.

Step 9. While still warm, roll in a cinnamon-and-sugar mixture, or cool and sprinkle with confectioners' sugar.

Nutritional content: Makes 12 servings (1 donut (48 g) per serving; includes 1 t. or 5 ml olive oil absorbed per donut, excludes toppings), Each serving contains: Calories (150); Total Fat (5 g); Saturated Fat (1 g); Cholesterol (15 mg); Sodium (100 mg); Potassium (31 mg); Total Carbohydrate (24 g); Dietary Fiber (1 g); Sugars (9 g); Protein (2 g). Nutrient(s) of note (percent of Daily Value): Iron 2%

Toppings, Sides, and Frostings

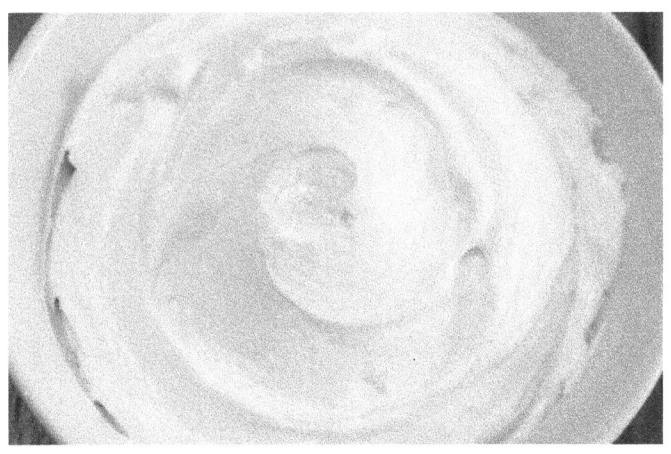

Cashew-Coconut Cream Topping

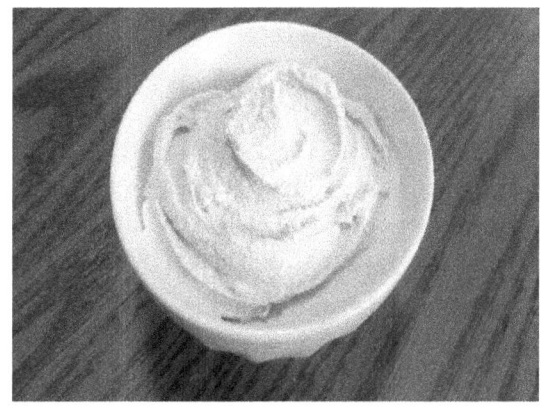

Use this sweet, creamy, and slightly tart topping in place of dairy-based whipped cream—it adds a nice finishing touch to cakes and pies. Be sure the raw cashews you use are gluten-free (many brands have inadvertently had gluten added during packaging and processing). For a creamier and less tart topping that is perfect as a filling in a layer cake, double the amount of coconut cream in step 3 and leave out the apple cider vinegar in Step 4. For a lighter whipped topping that is perfect on pies, follow the recipe for Whipped Coconut Cream on page 248. Makes about 1½ cups (360 g) of topping.

☑ **Allergy/Intolerance Substitutions:**

Corn: In step 4, use homemade confectioner's sugar made with tapioca starch (see page 70).

Coconut: Replace the coconut cream and coconut water in steps 3, 4, and 5 with your milk of choice. Add the milk in one-tablespoon (15 ml) increments as you may need less than the amount of coconut cream and water specified in the recipe below.

Tree nuts: Avoid this recipe or, if coconut is tolerated, make the Whipped Coconut Cream recipe on page 248.

☑ Reduced Sugar:
In step 4, leave out the confectioner's sugar, and either add 15 drops of clear, alcohol-free liquid stevia or leave out the stevia completely.

Topping Ingredients:
1½ c. raw cashews (225 g), soaked in water for a minimum of 2 hours
5 T. coconut cream (75 g)
½ t. clear vanilla extract (2.5 ml)
2 t. coconut water (10 ml)
2½ t. apple cider vinegar (12.5 ml)
2 T. confectioner's sugar (15 g)

Preparation the Night Before:
Place one 13.5-fluid-ounce (400 ml) can of coconut milk in the refrigerator. Do not use "lite" coconut milk.

Directions:
Step 1. Drain the raw cashews that have been soaking. Place them on a plate that has been lined with a paper towel, and blot dry.

Step 2. Place the cashews in a food processor, and pulse for one minute until the cashews reach a grainy consistency. Scrape the sides of the food processor bowl with a rubber spatula.

Step 3. Carefully open the can of coconut milk without shaking it or turning it upside-down. Add 5 T. (75 g) of the thick coconut cream (from the top of the can) to the food processor bowl, along with the clear vanilla extract and 1 teaspoon (5 ml) of coconut water (from the bottom of the can). Food process for 2 minutes, stopping the food processor once to scrape the sides of the bowl with a rubber spatula. Shut off the food processor.

Step 4. Add the second teaspoon (5 ml) of coconut water, the apple cider vinegar, and the confectioner's sugar. Food process 2 to 3 minutes more until a thick and creamy topping forms. Shut off the food processor.

Step 5. Scrape the sides of the bowl with a rubber spatula, and then food process for one more minute. If the topping is not creamy enough, mix in an additional teaspoon of coconut water and food process for one minute.

Step 6. Using the rubber spatula, remove the topping from the food processor bowl and place in a sealed glass container.

Step 7. Keep the topping at room temperature for use that day, or refrigerate for later use. Remove the container from the refrigerator 30 minutes before serving and remix if needed.

Nutritional content: Makes 12 servings (2 Tablespoons (25 g) per serving). Each serving contains: Calories (110); Total Fat (7 g); Saturated Fat (2 g); Cholesterol (0 mg); Sodium (5 mg); Potassium (10 mg); Total Carbohydrate (10 g); Dietary Fiber (1 g); Sugars (6 g); Protein (3 g). Nutrient(s) of note (percent of Daily Value): Calcium 2%, Iron 6%

Whipped Coconut Cream:

Refrigerate a 13.5-fluid-ounce (400-ml) can of full-fat coconut milk overnight. Place ⅔ cup (152 g) of the thick coconut cream from the can in a small metal mixing bowl; cover the bowl with plastic wrap and refrigerate for 1 hour or more (if using metal beaters for an electric mixer, refrigerate the beaters as well). (Note: if there is a layer of coconut oil on top of the cream in the can of coconut milk, scrape the oil off before measuring the coconut cream.) Twenty minutes before serving, remove the bowl from the refrigerator and peel off the plastic wrap. Add to the bowl 2 T. (15 g) confectioner's sugar, ½ t. (2.5 ml) vanilla extract, and ⅛ t. (0.6 g) cream of tartar. Beat till fluffy with an electric mixer (the coconut cream may be difficult to beat at first, but will loosen up after a minute). Scrape the sides of the bowl, and beat for one minute longer. Serve immediately. This cream can be covered, refrigerated, and stored for up to one week. Makes slightly less than 1 cup (167 g) of topping.

Chocolate Coconut Ganache or Frosting

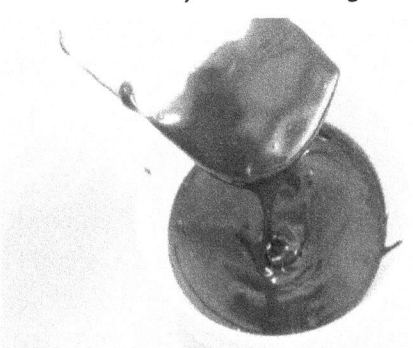

This easy-to-make ganache is rich and delicious, and can be used in several ways: serve the ganache warm as a "hot fudge" sauce (see photo); cool it to room temperature to use as a fudge-like icing; or beat in shortening to make a creamy frosting. Make sure the mixing bowl and rubber spatula used are completely dry before you start; even the slightest amount of water inadvertently added will ruin the consistency of the ganache. Store any leftover ganache in the refrigerator for up to two weeks; after storage, you will need to soften it in the microwave for about 15 seconds prior to use. Makes approximately 1½ cups (396 g) of ganache, enough for icing one cake layer; the frosting recipe makes 2 cups (480 g), enough for two layers.

☑ **Allergy/Intolerance Substitutions:**

Coconut: Avoid this recipe.

☑ **Reduced Sugar:**

None; this recipe does not work well with sugar-free chocolate chips.

Ganache Ingredients:
⅔ c. coconut cream (152 g) from one 13.5-fluid-ounce (400 ml) can of coconut milk (full fat)
10-oz. bag GF-DF-SF chocolate chips (283 g)
5 to 7 T. shortening (for frosting recipe only) (45 to 63 g)

Preparation the Night Before:
Place one 13.5-fluid-ounce (400 ml) can of coconut milk in the refrigerator. Do not use "lite" or homemade coconut milk.

Directions:
Step 1. Open the can of coconut milk without shaking it or turning it upside down. Remove ⅔ cup (152 g) of the thick cream at the top of the can and place it in a microwave-safe mixing bowl. Heat the coconut cream in the microwave for about 50 seconds.

Step 2. Add the chocolate chips. Stir with a rubber spatula till all of the chips are melted, and the ganache is smooth and glossy. If the chips still have not completely melted after stirring for one minute, microwave for 10 seconds more and mix again.

Step 3. Choose one of the variations below:
For warm ganache sauce: Let the ganache cool for 10 minutes. Pour it over ice cream or drizzle it over a slice of cake.

For ganache icing: Place a piece of plastic wrap directly on the surface of the ganache. Cool the ganache for about one hour at room temperature until it thickens (it should be thick but pourable). Remove the plastic wrap. Pour the ganache over a cake that has been removed from its pan and completely cooled, or drizzle it over cooled cookies. You can also spread the ganache over the top of a cooled cake that has not been removed from the pan (the ganache will form a thick, fudge-like layer on top). Place the frosted cake or cookies in a cool, dark room overnight to harden (do not refrigerate).

For frosting: Place a piece of plastic wrap directly on the surface of the ganache. Cool the ganache to room temperature for about two hours. Beat 5 T. (45 g) of shortening into the ganache for about one minute with an electric mixer till a smooth and creamy frosting forms. If the frosting is not thick enough, add the remaining 2 T. (18 g) of shortening and beat in. Scrape the sides of the bowl with a rubber spatula. Beat for one minute more with the electric mixer till the frosting is smooth, thick, and uniform in color. Slather on a cooled cake or cookies with an offset spatula or knife. Place the frosted cake or cookies in a cool, dark room overnight to harden (do not refrigerate).

Nutritional content (ganache): Makes 12 servings (2 Tablespoons (40 g) per serving). Each serving contains: Calories (160); Total Fat (7 g); Saturated Fat (5 g); Cholesterol (0 mg); Sodium (5 mg); Potassium (150 mg); Total Carbohydrate (25 g); Dietary Fiber (0 g); Sugars (22 g); Protein (1 g). Nutrient(s) of note (percent of Daily Value): Calcium 4%, Iron 6%

Nutritional content (frosting): Makes 16 servings (2 Tablespoons (36 g) per serving). Each serving contains: Calories (170); Total Fat (11 g); Saturated Fat (6 g); Cholesterol (0 mg); Sodium (5 mg); Potassium (113 mg); Total Carbohydrate (19 g); Dietary Fiber (0 g); Sugars (16 g); Protein (1 g). Nutrient(s) of note (percent of Daily Value): Calcium 2%, Iron 4%

Vanilla Frosting

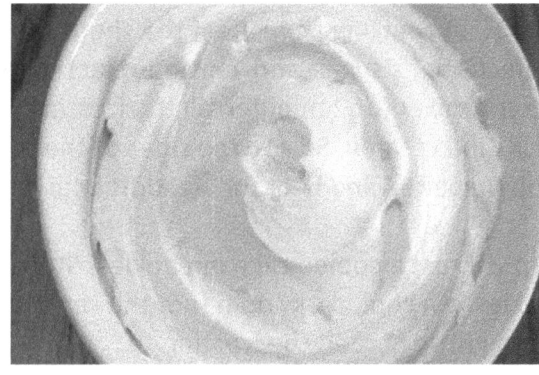

This frosting is thick, flavorful, and rich. For icings with different flavors, replace the vanilla extract with a different extract (e.g., orange or raspberry). For the whitest frosting, use a shortening that is pure white in color. If you would like a color other than white, add a few drops of GF-DF-SF food color as you mix the frosting. If you tolerate dairy, you can exchange the shortening for butter, but the frosting will be a cream color instead of white. Makes approximately 1½ cups (360 g) of frosting, enough for one cake layer.

☑ Allergy/Intolerance Substitutions:
Corn: In step 1, use homemade confectioner's sugar made with tapioca starch (see page 70; this frosting may be slightly gritty if homemade confectioner's sugar is used).

☑ Reduced Sugar:
No suggestions given; this recipe does not work well without the sugar.

Frosting Ingredients:
1 c. shortening (144 g)
⅔ c. confectioner's sugar (88 g)
½ t. vanilla extract (2.5 ml)

Directions:
Step 1. In a mixing bowl, beat the shortening, confectioner's sugar, and vanilla extract together with an electric mixer for 2 minutes till the frosting is smooth, thick, and creamy. Scrape the sides of the bowl with a rubber spatula and beat for an additional minute.

Step 2. Frost a cooled cake or cookies. Store the cake or cookies in a cool, dark room (not the refrigerator) overnight to harden the frosting.

Step 3. Store any unused frosting in a sealed glass container in the refrigerator for up to two weeks. Bring back to room temperature before using.

Nutritional content: Makes 12 servings (2 Tablespoons (24 g) per serving). Each serving contains: Calories (170); Total Fat (17 g); Saturated Fat (8 g); Cholesterol (0 mg); Sodium (0 mg); Potassium (0 mg); Total Carbohydrate (7 g); Dietary Fiber (0 g); Sugars (6 g); Protein (0 g). Nutrient(s) of note (percent of Daily Value): none

Lemon-, Orange-, or Vanilla-Flavored Icing

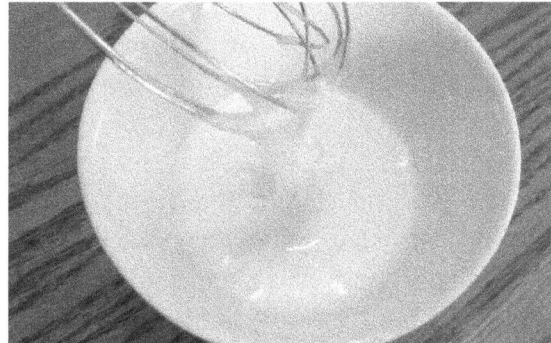

Try drizzling this icing over crumb cakes and muffins, or slather it on cookies. Extract flavorings besides lemon, orange, and vanilla can be used as well. This recipe makes about ¼ cup (74 g) of icing, enough to drizzle on one cake or to frost about 12 cookies (double the recipe for more cookies).

☑ Allergy/Intolerance Substitutions:
Corn: Use homemade confectioner's sugar made with tapioca starch (see page 70).

☑ Reduced Sugar:
No suggestions given; this recipe does not work well without the confectioners' sugar.

Icing Ingredients:
½ c. confectioners' sugar (60 g), sifted
½ t. lemon, orange, or vanilla extract (2.5 ml)
2 t. water (10 ml)

Directions:
Step 1. Place the ingredients in a small mixing bowl. With a rubber spatula, mix together the confectioners' sugar, extract, and water till a smooth icing forms. Mix in 1 to 2 drops of GF-DF-SF food coloring if a color other than white is desired.

Step 2. Test the icing for thickness before use. For frosting cookies, the icing should go on thick, should not drip down the sides of the cookies, and should smooth out in appearance after it sits on the cookies for a minute. For drizzling on cakes and muffins, the icing should slowly flow off of a spoon in a thin stream. If the icing is too thick, mix in ¼ t. (1 ml) water and stir; if the icing is too runny, mix in ½ t. (1.5 g) confectioners' sugar. Repeat as needed till the desired consistency is achieved.

Step 3. Immediately drizzle on cooled muffins or cakes, or slather on cooled cookies. Decorate with GF-DF-SF sprinkles (optional) before the icing hardens (this icing hardens quickly at room temperature).

Nutritional content: Makes 12 servings (1 teaspoon (6 g) per serving). Each serving contains: Calories (20); Total Fat (0 g); Saturated Fat (0 g); Cholesterol (0 mg); Sodium (0 mg); Potassium (0 mg); Total Carbohydrate (5 g); Dietary Fiber (0 g); Sugars (5 g); Protein (0 g). Nutrient(s) of note (percent of Daily Value): none

Frozen Coconut Vanilla Custard

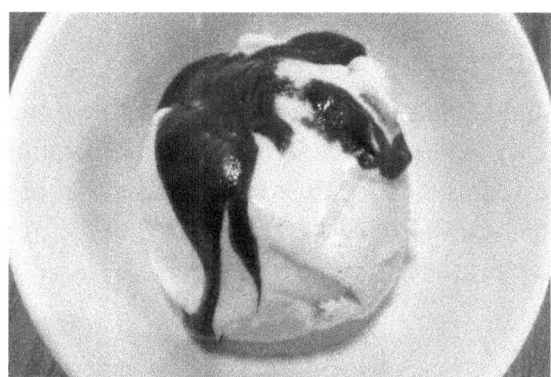

There's nothing like fresh, homemade ice cream! The vanilla bean adds just the right amount of vanilla flavor to this recipe. The basic recipe is delicious as is, but you can add shaved chocolate or small chunks of fruit if you like during the freezing process. I like to serve this frozen custard with warm Chocolate Coconut Ganache (see photo insert and recipe on page 249). Start this recipe well in advance of serving it, since the custard mixture needs to be chilled for at least two hours before freezing it into ice cream (unless you have an ice cream maker with a compressor). This recipe is somewhat labor-intensive, but well worth the effort! Makes approximately 3 cups (552 g).

☑ Allergy/Intolerance Substitutions:
Coconut: Avoid this recipe.
Eggs: Avoid this recipe.

☑ Other Warning:
High in saturated fat from coconut.

☑ Reduced Sugar:
In step 3, replace the honey with 40 drops of clear, alcohol-free liquid stevia.

Custard Ingredients:
Two 13.5-fluid-ounce (400 ml) cans of coconut milk (do not use "lite" or homemade coconut milk)
4 large egg yolks
¼ c. honey (87 g)
1 vanilla bean pod

Directions:
Step 1. Place the freeze-able canister of your ice cream maker in the freezer the day before beginning this recipe (skip this step for ice cream makers that use a salt-and-ice mixture to freeze the cream, or that have an electric compressor).

Step 2. Pour the two cans of coconut milk into a medium-sized saucepan. Warm the coconut milk over medium heat, stirring constantly with a heat-resistant rubber spatula to prevent it from sticking to the bottom of the pan. Once the coconut milk begins to steam slightly (the temperature will be about 135° F/57° C), turn off the heat.

Step 3. In a large mixing bowl, whisk together the egg yolks and honey till the mixture is slightly frothy.

Step 4. Remove about ¼ cup (59 ml) of the steaming coconut milk from the sauce pan and *slowly* pour it into the egg mixture, whisking the eggs as you pour. Continue whisking for about 30 seconds. Pour a little more of the coconut milk into the eggs, and continue whisking. Continue to slowly add the coconut milk to the eggs (while whisking) until half of the coconut milk has been added. Pour the egg and milk mixture (i.e., the custard) back into the saucepan, whisking the mixture in the sauce pan as you pour.

Step 5. Slice open the vanilla bean and scrape out the seeds. Add both the seeds and the vanilla bean pod to the custard and stir.

Step 6. Heat the custard gradually over medium-low heat, *stirring constantly* with a heat-resistant rubber spatula and scraping the bottom of the pan, until it thickens (20 to 30 minutes) and reaches a temperature of about 180° to 190° F (82° to 88° C). If the mixture starts to bubble as it is being thickened, turn the heat down to low. If lumps begin to form, remove the pan from the heat immediately. A simple test for knowing if the custard has adequately thickened is to dip the rubber spatula into the custard, cool the custard on the spatula for several seconds, and then draw a line through the custard on the spatula with a fingertip (make sure the custard has adequately cooled before you do this); if the edges of the line remain sharp and do not drip together after five seconds, you know the custard has adequately thickened. It is important to not rush the cooking of the custard; the longer it cooks, the less water it will contain, creating a creamier frozen custard.

Step 7. Remove the vanilla bean pod from the custard. Pour the custard into a medium-sized bowl. Place a sheet of plastic wrap over the custard (the plastic wrap should be in direct contact with the surface of the custard). Refrigerate for a minimum of 2 hours (or less if your ice cream maker has an electric compressor).
Step 8. Follow the directions for your ice cream maker to freeze the custard. After it is frozen, scrape the ice cream out of the canister and enjoy. Store the ice cream in a sealed container in the freezer.

Nutritional content: Makes 6 servings (½ cup (157 g) per serving). Each serving contains: Calories (340); Total Fat (31 g); Saturated Fat (26 g); Cholesterol (125 mg); Sodium (25 mg); Potassium (309 mg); Total Carbohydrate (15 g); Dietary Fiber (0 g); Sugars (11 g); Protein (5 g). Nutrient(s) of note (percent of Daily Value): Vitamin A 4%, Calcium 4%, Vitamin C 2%, Iron 25%

Coconut Yogurt

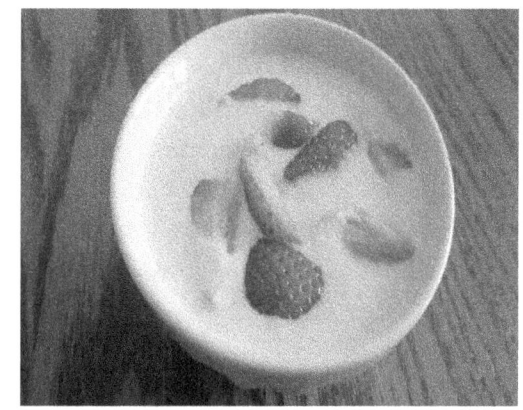

*F**inding a yogurt in the store that is both reasonably priced and free of gluten, dairy, and soy can be difficult. Making your own yogurt is easy and less expensive, but you will need a yogurt maker to proceed (preferably one with individual yogurt jars). This recipe calls for coconut butter (also called creamed coconut or cream of coconut) as the main ingredient; using coconut butter that comes in a 7-ounce (200 g) box is usually less expensive than using coconut butter that comes in a jar. The coconut butter yields a thick yogurt with a slightly gritty texture. For a smoother but more liquid yogurt, replace the coconut butter and water in the recipe with 6 cups of coconut milk. Because this yogurt is high in calories and saturated fat, you may wish to eat only 3 oz. (about ⅓ cup or 85 g) at any one time. Be sure to consult your doctor or nutritionist before introducing this yogurt into your diet because of the saturated fat and the live bacterial cultures it contains. This recipe makes a total of 6 cups (1488 g) of yogurt.*

Finding a Yogurt Starter:
True yogurt contains two main types of bacteria: *Lactobacillus bulgaricus* and *Streptococcus thermophilus*[66] (some brands of yogurt contain other strains of bacteria as well). Finding a GF-DF-SF starter mix that contains these two strains of bacteria (e.g., belle+bella™ brand) is key to making an authentic yogurt. Once you have created a batch of yogurt using the yogurt starter, reserve half of a jar of the yogurt to use as the starter for your next batch of yogurt. You can also purchase a container of plain GF-DF-SF yogurt from the store to use as the starter. The honey included in this recipe provides the sugar needed to feed the bacteria during the incubation process.

If you have difficulty finding a GF-DF-SF yogurt starter, probiotic capsules can be used instead (note: using probiotics is not recommended since they usually contain additional strains of bacteria which will incubate in your yogurt along with the two desired strains of bacteria). If you do decide to use probiotic capsules as the starter, you may need to use two different kinds of capsules in order to include the two types of bacteria found in yogurt. Check the labels on the probiotic bottles to see if the *Lactobacillus bulgaricus* and *Streptococcus thermophilus* bacteria are included. Also make sure that the probiotics are free of gluten, dairy, and soy, and processed in a gluten-free facility (a recent Columbia University Medical Center study found that 55% of the probiotics tested contained gluten, although most were under the 20 ppm required by the FDA for gluten-free food labeling[67]). Finally, check with your medical practitioner to make sure the strains of bacteria in the probiotics you choose are suited to your health concerns.

☑ Allergy/Intolerance Substitutions:
Corn: Use a probiotic or yogurt starter that does not contain corn starch and that is not derived from corn (corn may be listed as an inactive ingredient).
Coconut: Avoid this recipe.
Bovine/porcine: Leave out the gelatin, or replace with agar powder.

☑ Other Warnings:
Contains live bacterial cultures.
High in saturated fat from coconut.

☑ Reduced Sugar:
No suggestions given; the honey is needed to feed the bacteria during the incubation process. Trace amounts of the sugars in the honey may remain in the finished yogurt.

Yogurt Ingredients:
One 16 oz. jar (453 g) or three 7 oz. (200 g) boxes of
    creamed coconut or coconut butter
Filtered or purified water
1 T. honey (22 g)
1 to 2 packets of GF-DF-SF yogurt starter, or 2 T. (32 g)
    plain GF-DF-SF yogurt
1 t. unflavored, powdered gelatin or agar (2.5 g)

Directions:

Step 1. Open the jar or boxes of coconut butter. A white layer of coconut oil will likely have formed on top of the cream-colored coconut butter; you will need to remove this layer of oil before making the yogurt. For the boxed coconut cream, simply cut off the 1-inch-thick (2.5-cm-thick) layer of oil. The oil layer is usually thinner in jarred coconut butter, and can usually be scraped off with a knife or spoon. Reserve the coconut oil in a separate jar for other recipes.

Step 2. Chop the coconut butter into small cubes, roughly the size of a pea. Place the chopped coconut butter in a 2-quart (1.9 liter) or larger glass measuring cup. Fill the measuring cup with the filtered water till the coconut butter and water mixture measures 6 cups (1.4 liters) total.

Step 3. Pour the water and coconut butter into a medium-sized sauce pan. Heat the coconut and water mixture on medium heat, stirring constantly with a heat-resistant rubber spatula, till the cubes of coconut butter melt completely into the water, and the temperature of the mixture reaches 130° F or 54° C. Turn off the burner.

Step 4. Mix in the honey. Pour the coconut mixture back into the 2-quart (1.9 liter) glass measuring cup.

Step 5. Stir the mixture to bring its temperature down to between 110° and 115° F (43° to 46° C). Pour about 4 fluid ounces (118 ml) of the mixture into one of the yogurt maker jars. To this jar, add the yogurt starter (follow the manufacturer's instructions on the yogurt starter package in order to determine the correct amount to add) or add the 2 T. (32 g) of GF-DF-SF plain yogurt; if using probiotic capsules, pull the capsules apart and add only the powder. Using a narrow rubber spatula, mix the starter into the 4 oz. (118 ml) of coconut mixture for one to two minutes until it is *completely* combined. Pour the jar of the coconut/starter mixture back into the 2-quart (1.9 liter) measuring cup with the rest of the coconut mixture, and mix thoroughly.

Step 6. Dissolve the teaspoon of gelatin or agar in 2 Tablespoons (30 ml) of warm water in a separate bowl or cup. Immediately pour the gelatin or agar mixture into the coconut/starter mixture and stir well.

Step 7. Pour the coconut/starter mixture into each of the yogurt maker jars, dividing it equally between jars. Put the lids on the filled jars, and place them into the yogurt maker. Set the timer on the yogurt maker for 15 hours or more (the longer you cook the yogurt, the thicker and more tart it will be; 15 hours is a good length of time for your first batch of yogurt). Push the "start" button.

Step 8. After the yogurt has finished incubating for 15 hours, place the yogurt maker jars in the refrigerator and chill for at least 6 hours. If a thin layer of liquid forms on top of the yogurt, either pour it off or mix it back into the yogurt before serving.

Nutritional content: Makes 16 servings (3 oz. (39 g) per serving). Each serving contains: Calories (260); Total Fat (26 g); Saturated Fat (23 g); Cholesterol (0 mg); Sodium (15 mg); Potassium (206 mg); Total Carbohydrate (9 g); Dietary Fiber (0 g); Sugars (1 g); Protein (2 g). Nutrient(s) of note (percent of Daily Value): Iron 6%

References

1. USDA, "Food Composition," National Agricultural Food Library, http://fnic.nal.usda.gov/food-composition (accessed 15 May, 2015).

2. SELF Nutrition Data, "Arrowroot, flour," http://nutritiondata.self.com/facts/cereal-grains-and-pasta/5677/2 (accessed 8 February, 2016).

3. Nutrition-and-you.com, "Arrowroot Nutrition Facts," http://www.nutrition-and-you.com/arrowroot.html (accessed 8 February, 2016).

4. Advameg, Inc., "Baking Soda," *How Products Are Made*, http://www.madehow.com/Volume-1/Baking-Soda.html (accessed 1 Nov. 2014).

5. SELF Nutrition Data, "Rice Flour, Brown," http://nutritiondata.self.com (accessed 15 Nov. 2014).

6. George Mateljan Foundation, "Brown Rice," http://www.whfoods.com/genpage.php?tname=foodspice&dbid=128 (accessed 1 Nov. 2014).

7. Consumer Reports, "How Much Arsenic Is in Your Rice?," http://www.consumerreports.org/cro/magazine/2015/01/how-much-arsenic-is-in-your-rice/index.htm (accessed 11 Oct. 2016).

8. U. S. Food and Drug Administration, "FDA Statement on Testing and Analysis of Arsenic in Rice and Rice Products," http://www.fda.gov/Food/FoodborneIllnessContaminants/Metals/ucm367263.htm (accessed 11 Oct. 2016).

9. GuarGum.biz, "Guar Gum Manufacturing Process," http://www.guargum.biz/guargum_manufacturing_process.html (accessed 1 Nov. 2014).

10. SELF Nutrition Data, "Millet, Raw," http://nutritiondata.self.com (accessed 15 Nov. 2014).

11. George Mateljan Foundation, "Millet," http://www.whfoods.com/genpage.php?tname=foodspice&dbid=53#historyuse (accessed 1 Nov. 2014).

12. Marie Dannie, "Nutritional Value of Potato Starch & Corn Starch," http://www.livestrong.com/article/545501-nutritional-value-of-potato-starch-corn-starch (accessed 1 Feb. 2016).

13. SELF Nutrition Data, "Rice Flour, White," http://nutritiondata.self.com (accessed 15 Nov. 2014).

14. SELF Nutrition Data, "Sorghum," http://nutritiondata.self.com (accessed 15 November, 2014).

15. Gramene, "Sorghum Introduction," http://www.gramene.org/species/sorghum/sorghum_intro.html (accessed 1 Nov. 2014).

16. SELF Nutrition Data, "Tapioca Starch," http://nutritiondata.self.com/facts/custom/1275851/1 (accessed 8 February, 2016).

17. Wikipedia, "Tapioca," https://en.wikipedia.org/wiki/Tapioca (accessed 8 February, 2016).

18. WiseGEEK, "What is Xanthan Gum?, "http://www.wisegeek.com/what-is-xanthan-gum.htm#didyouknowout (accessed 1 Nov. 2014).

19. Sylvie Tremblay, "Almond Meal Nutrition," Livestrong.com, http://www.livestrong.com/article/113190-almond-meal-nutrition/ (accessed 9 Nov. 2014).

20. Nutfarm, "Almond History," http://www.nutsforalmonds.com/history.htm (accessed 9 Nov. 2014).

21. SELF Nutrition Data, "Seeds, Chia Seeds, Dried Nutrition Facts & Calories," http://nutritiondata.self.com/facts/nut-and-seed-products/3061/2 (accessed 11 Oct. 2016).

22. Kerry Neville, "Chia Seeds: Tiny Seeds with a Rich History," Food & Nutrition Magazine, http://www.foodandnutrition.org/January-

February-2014/Chia-Seeds-Tiny-Seeds-with-a-Rich-History (accessed 11 Oct. 2016).

23. SELF Nutrition Data, "Nuts, Coconut Milk, Raw (Liquid Expressed from Grated Meat and Water)," http://nutritiondata.self.com/facts/nut-and-seed-products/3113/2 (accessed 9 Nov. 2014).

24. Umesh Rudrappa, "Coconut Nutrition Facts," http://www.nutrition-and-you.com/coconut.html (accessed 9 Nov. 2014).

25. WiseGEEK, "What is Coconut Cream?," http://www.wisegeek.com/what-is-coconut-cream.htm (accessed 9 Nov. 2014).

26. Umesh Rudrappa, "Coconut Nutrition Facts," http://www.nutrition-and-you.com/coconut.html (accessed 9 Nov. 2014).

27. SELF Nutrition Data, "Egg, Whole, Raw, Fresh," http://nutritiondata.self.com/facts/dairy-and-egg-products/111/2 (accessed 15 Nov. 2014).

28. Francisco Lopez-Jimenez, "Eggs: Are they good or bad for my cholesterol?," Mayo Clinic, http://www.mayoclinic.org/diseases-conditions/high-blood-cholesterol/expert-answers/cholesterol/faq-20058468 (accessed 26 July 2017).

29. SELF Nutrition Data, "Seeds, Flaxseed Nutrition Facts & Calories," http:// http://nutritiondata.self.com/facts/nut-and-seed-products/3163/2 (accessed 11 Oct. 2016).

30. North Dakota State University, "A Flax Timeline: A Brief History of Flax from 8000 BCE to Present Day," https://www.ag.ndsu.edu/ccv/flax/history-and-uses-1 (accessed 11 Oct. 2016).

31. SELF Nutrition Data, "Honey," http://nutritiondata.self.com/facts/sweets/5568/2 (accessed 8 February, 2016).

32. Suzanne S. Wiley, "Types of Sugars in Honey," Livestrong.com, http://www.livestrong.com/article/260781-types-of-sugars-in-honey (accessed 9 Nov. 2014).

33. Dr. Andrew Weil, "Is lard healthy?," https://www.drweil.com/diet-nutrition/nutrition/is-lard-healthy(accessed 10August 2017).

34. Ibid.

35. George Mateljan Foundation, "Oats," http://www.whfoods.com/genpage.php?tname=nutrientprofile&dbid=109 (accessed 1 Nov. 2014).

36. Lance Gibson and Garren Benson, "Origin, History, and Uses of Oat (*Avena sativa*) and Wheat (*Triticumaestivum*)," Iowa State University, http://agron-www.agron.iastate.edu/Courses/agron212/Readings/Oat_wheat_history.htm (accessed 1 Nov. 2014).

37. SELF Nutrition Data, "Oil, Olive, Salad or Cooking," http://nutritiondata.self.com/facts/fats-and-oils/509/2 (accessed 8 February, 2016).

38. Dr. Axe, "8 Quinoa Nutrition Facts & Benefits, Including Weight Loss," Dr. Axe Food and Medicine, https://draxe.com/10-quinoa-nutrition-facts-benefits (accessed 3 September, 2017).

39. Ancient Grains, "Quinoa history and origin," http://www.ancientgrains.com/quinoa-history-and-origin, (accessed 3 September, 2017).

40. Dr. Axe, "8 Quinoa Nutrition Facts & Benefits, Including Weight Loss," Dr. Axe Food and Medicine, https://draxe.com/10-quinoa-nutrition-facts-benefits (accessed 3 September, 2017).

41. Clay McNight, "Why is Hydrogenated Oil Bad for You?," Livestrong.com, http://www.livestrong.com/article/272066-why-is-hydrogenated-oil-bad-for-you/ (accessed 9 Nov. 2014).

42. Natalie DigateMuth, "The Truth About Stevia—The So-called "Healthy" Alternative Sweetener," Certified News, https://www.acefitness.org/certifiednewsarticle/1644/the-truth-about-stevia-the-so-called-quot-healthy/ (accessed 2 January 2016).

43. Essortment, "History of Sugar," http://www.essortment.com/history-sugar-41718.html (accessed 9 Nov. 2014).

44. Livestrong.com, "How is Sucrose Digested?," http://www.livestrong.com/article/316805-how-is-sucrose-digested/ (accessed 8 February, 2016).

45. U.S. Department of Health and Human Services, "A food labeling guide," https://www.fda.gov/downloads/food/guidanceregulation/ucm265446.pdf (accessed 28 July, 2017).

46. US Food and Drug Administration, " 'Gluten-Free' Now Means What It Says," http://www.fda.gov/ForConsumers/ConsumerUpdates/ucm363069.htm (accessed 15 November, 2014).

47. "What is casein?," Peas and Figs, http://www.peasandfigs.co.uk/intolerances/casein-free/ (accessed 10 August 2017).

48. Chris Kresser, "Harmful or harmless: Soy lecithin," Let's Take Back Your Health—Starting Now, https://chriskresser.com/harmful-or-harmless-soy-lecithin (accessed 10 August 2017).

49. AllergyAdvisor.com, "Hidden allergens in foods," http://allergyadvisor.com/hidden2.htm (accessed 26 July 2017).

50. AllergyAdvisor.com, "Hidden allergens in foods," http://allergyadvisor.com/hidden.htm (accessed 26 July 2017).

51. Mariska de Wild-Scholten, "From Too Much Histamine to Too Much Migraine," *Too Much Magazine*, http://toomuchmag.com/from-too-much-histamine-to-too-much-migraine/ (accessed 5 Dec. 2015).

52. Dr. Janice Jonega, "Histamine Intolerance," Foods Matter.com, http://www.foodsmatter.com/allergy_intolerance/histamine/articles/histamine_joneja.html (accessed 5 Dec. 2015).

53. "Histamine Potential of Foods and Additives," www.histaminintoleranz.ch (accessed 21 Jan. 2016).

54. Ibid.

55. Dr. Janice Jonega, "Histamine Intolerance," Foods Matter.com, http://www.foodsmatter.com/allergy_intolerance/histamine/articles/histamine_joneja.html (accessed 5 Dec. 2015).

56. "Histamine Potential of Foods and Additives," www.histaminintoleranz.ch (accessed 21 Jan. 2016).

57. Melissa Lind, "Nightshade Vegetables and Arthritis Pain," Livestrong.com, http://www.livestrong.com/article/431059-nightshade-vegetables-and-arthritis-pain (accessed 15 Nov. 2014).

58. "Salicylate Sensitivity," Salicylatesensitivity.com, http://salicylatesensitivity.com/about/food-guide (accessed 8 June, 2017).

59. Christine Sexton, "Salicylate intolerance: The complete guide," Diet vs. Disease, https://www.dietvsdisease.org/salicylate-intolerance/ (accessed online 31 July 2017).

60. "Salicylate in food," Food Can Make You Ill, http://www.foodcanmakeyouill.co.uk/salicylate-in-food.html (accessed online 31 July, 2017).

61. Mari J. Dionne, "The oxalates and salicylates food list," PK Diet.com, http://www.pkdiet.com/pdf/oxalate%20lists.pdf (accessed online 31 July, 2017).

62. "Nutrition Guide for Fructose Malabsorption," HealthHype.com, http://www.healthhype.com/nutrition-guide-for-fructose-malabsorption.html (accessed 1 January 2016).

63. U.S. Department of Health and Human Services, "A food labeling guide," https://www.fda.gov/downloads/food/guidanceregulation/ucm265446.pdf (accessed 28 July, 2017).

64. Anthony Samsel and Stephanie Seneff, 2013, "Glyphosate, pathways to modern diseases II: Celiac sprue and gluten intolerance," *Interdisciplinary Toxicology*, 6(4), 159-185.

65. "Substitution Solutions," *Living Without's: Gluten-free & More Magazine*, June/July 2015, p. 109.

66. Breaking the Vicious Cycle, "Yoghurt - What Kind of Yoghurt Starter to Use," http://www.breakingtheviciouscycle.info/

knowledge_base/detail/yoghurt-what-kind-of-yoghurt-starter-to-use/ (accessed 15 Nov. 2014).

67. Alexandra Sifferlin, "Many Probiotics Contain Traces of Gluten, Study Says," *Time*, http://time.com/3860361/probiotics-gluten/ (accessed 4 June 2015).

Index

Abbreviations	14
Allergen product labelling	42
All-but-the-kitchen-sink Bars	219
Almond meal	30
Apple Oat Muffins	95
Applesauce-Oat Sandwich Bread	125
Arrowroot starch	23
Baking powder	31
Baking soda	24
Baking tips	46
Banana Pecan Chocolate Chip Waffles	90
Banana Chip Bread	105
Basic Dinner Biscuits	169
Basil's Chocolate Biscotti	231
Batter-dipped Fried Food	86
Biscuits	169, 173
Blueberry Crumb Cake	147
Blueberry Custard Pie Filling	194
Blueberry Muffins	150
Blueberry Scones	181
Breads	103
Breakfast Cookies	91
Brown rice flour	24
Brownies	227
"Butter" Cookies	235

Cakes	133
Cane-sugar-free Fruit Pie	200
Carrot Spice Bread	117
Cashew-Coconut Cream Topping	245
Celiac Disease	43
Chia seeds	31
Chia Seed Egg Replacer	73
Chocolate Chip Cake	155
Chocolate Chip Cookie Cups	206
Chocolate Chip Cookies	203
Chocolate Coconut Ganache or Frosting	249
Coconut allergies	64
Coconut milk	32, 70
Coconut Yogurt	261
Confectioner's sugar	70
Cookies and Treats	201
Corn Bread with a Kick	121
Corn allergies	53
Cranberry Orange Scones	177
Dairy product labelling	44
Disclaimer	8
Do-It-Yourself ingredients	70
Double-crust Pie Dough	195
Easy Breakfast Recipes	77
Egg-related concerns	54
Egg replacers	73
Eggs	33

Faux Double-crust Pie	200
Flax meal	34
Flax Meal Egg Replacer	73
Flour storage	51
Flour substitutions	66
Fresh Strawberry Cake	159
Fried Dough	239
Fritters	85
Frostings	249, 253
Frozen Coconut Vanilla Custard	257
Fruit and Vegetable Breads	103
Gluten-free Flour Mix Recipe	19
Gluten product labelling	43
Gingerbread Cookies	215
Granola	79
Guar gum	25
Histamine intolerance	20, 54
Home-style Poultry Stuffing	129
Honey	35
Honey & Spice Cookies	211
Ice cream (frozen custard)	257
Icings	255
Kitchen preparation	49
Lard	36
Lemon Almond Muffins	99
Lemon-, Orange-, or Vanilla-flavored Icing	255
Maple Berry Crunch	163

Millet flour	26
Milk of choice	36
Moist Almond Crumb Cake	143
Muffins	95, 99, 150
Nightshade (tomato) sensitivities	58
Non-rising Egg Replacer	76
Not-so-plain Sugar Cookies	207
Nut milks	71
Nutrition analysis	8
Oats	37
Oil sensitivities	58
Old-fashioned Oatmeal Cookies	223
Olive oil	38, 58
Pancakes	83
Peach Upside-down Cake	151
Peanut allergies	59
Pie doughs	189, 195
Pizza Dough	185
Potato starch	26
Pumpkin Bread	109
Quinoa flour	39
References	267
Rice	59
Rice allergies	20, 59
Rice milk	72
Rich Chocolate Cake	139
Rising Egg Replacer	74
Rosemary-Garlic Biscuits	173

Salicylate intolerance	20, 60
Seed meals	72
Shortening	39, 58
Simple Yellow Cake	135
Single-crust Pie Dough	189
Sorghum flour	28
Soy product labelling	45
Stevia	40, 64
Storing gluten-free flours	51
Sugar (refined cane)	41
Sugar concerns	63
Super Rich Brownies	227
Sweet rice flour	27
Tapioca starch	28
Tree nut allergies	64
Vanilla frosting	253
Waffles	87
Whipped Coconut Cream	248
Xanthan Gum	20, 29
Yogurt	261
Zucchini Bread	113